Gynaecological and Obstetric Pathology for the MRCOG

Proposed titles in the MRCOG Series

Antenatal Disorders for the MRCOG

Contraception for the MRCOG

Genetics and Fetal Medicine for the MRCOG

Gynaecological Oncology for the MRCOG

Gynaecological Pathology for the MRCOG

Gynaecological Urology for the MRCOG

Infertility for the MRCOG

Intrapartum Care for the MRCOG

Menstrual Problems for the MRCOG

Neonatology for the MRCOG

Reproductive Endocrinology for the MRCOG

The MRCOG: A Guide to the Examination

Gynaecological and Obstetric Pathology for the MRCOG

Harold Fox

MD, FRCPath, FRCOG, Emeritus Professor of Reproductive Pathology, Department of Pathological Sciences, University of Manchester, Stopford Building, Oxford Road, Manchester, M13 9PT

C. Hilary Buckley

MD, FRCPath, Reader in Gynaecological Pathology, Department of Reproductive Pathology, St. Mary's Hospital, Whitworth Park, Manchester M13 0JH

With a chapter on Cervical Cytology
by Professor Dulcie V. Coleman

MD, FRCPath, Professor of Cell Pathology, Department of Cytopathology and Cytogenetics, St. Mary's Hospital, Praed Street, London W2 1NY

Series Editor: Peter Milton

MD, FRCOG, Consultant Obstetrician and Gynaecologist
Addenbrooke's and Rosie Maternity Hospital, Robinson Way, Cambridge CB2 2SW

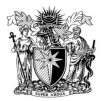

RCOG Press

Published by the **RCOG Press** at the
Royal College of Obstetricians and Gynaecologists
27 Sussex Place, Regent's Park
London NW1 4RG

Registered Charity No. 213280

Cover Illustration: A cytologist using the PapNet® Testing System. Reproduced by kind permission of Neuromedical Systems Incorporated.

Designed by Geoffrey Wadsley
Printed by Latimer Trend & Co Ltd, Plymouth

Acknowledgements

Figures 8.6–8.10 are reproduced from Fox, H. *Pathology of the Placenta*, 2nd edition 1997, by kind permission of WB Saunders Ltd. Figures 4.17–4.21 are reproduced from Buckley, C. H. and Fox, H. *Biopsy Pathology of the Endometrium*, 1989, by kind permission of Chapman and Hall, London. The remaining figures in Chapters 1–8 are reproduced from Fox, H. and Buckley, C. H. 'The female genital tract and ovaries' in McGee, J. O'D., Isaacson, P. G. and Wright, N. A. (Eds) *Oxford Textbook of Pathology*, 1992, by kind permission of Oxford University Press. Figures 9.1 and 9.2 were kindly provided by Dr Margherita Branca, Instituto Superiore di Sanita, Rome. Figure 9.19 is reproduced by kind permission of Neuromedical Systems Incorporated. Table 9.3 is reproduced by kind permission of Oxford University Press.

Contents

Preface   vi

1   The vulva   1

2   The vagina   19

3   The cervix   25

4   The endometrium   45

5   The myometrium   71

6   The fallopian tube   77

7   The ovary   87

8   Abnormalities related to pregnancy   127

9   Cervical cytology   143
    Professor Dulcie V. Coleman

    Suggested references for further reading   171

    Index   173

Preface

Possession of the MRCOG is an essential prerequisite for higher training within our specialty, both in the United Kingdom and in many countries overseas – the MRCOG has a high standing not only in the UK and the Commonwealth but increasingly within Europe. At the present time there are Fellows and Members of our College in over 80 countries throughout the world and the number of candidates taking the MRCOG examination continues to rise.

Preparing for the examination involves not only working in carefully monitored training posts but also a substantial amount of academic preparation and, from 1998, the submission of a 5000–8000 word dissertation on an obstetric or gynaecological topic.

In carrying out such studies candidates have traditionally used major standard works ranging from 'Jeffcoate's' and 'Donald' in my days during the 1970s to the present large, excellent, multi-author textbooks.

Whatever the clinical problem being studied, a thorough understanding of the background anatomy, physiology, histology and pathology is essential. This concise and beautifully illustrated volume will, I am sure, be used as an invaluable revision text by candidates preparing for the Part I and Part II MRCOG Examination, and also as a readily accessible, succinct, and up-to-date reference text by practising clinicians.

Peter Milton
RCOG Publications Committee 1992–96
June 1998

1 The vulva

Dermatological disorders

The vulvar skin is part of the body integument and is therefore subject to all the disorders that can affect the skin elsewhere; for example, lichen planus, psoriasis, or pemphigus. Lichen simplex and lichen sclerosus do, however, merit special attention, partly because they occur with some frequency in the skin of the vulva and partly because these two disorders have until recently been regarded, rather illogically, as falling into a separate category of 'vulvar dystrophies', a form of nomenclature now obsolete.

LICHEN SIMPLEX

Previously classed as 'hyperplastic dystrophy', lichen simplex appears as circumscribed areas of thickened red or white skin, usually on the labia majora. Histologically, the squamous epithelium is thickened, and shows acanthosis, elongation of the rete pegs, parakeratosis and hyperkeratosis. Figure 1.1 shows a non-specific chronic inflammatory cell infiltrate of the dermis. In the absence of a dermal inflammatory infiltrate, the lesion is simply classed as 'squamous hyperplasia'. Lichen simplex is not associated with any increased risk of vulvar carcinoma.

LICHEN SCLEROSUS

This condition can occur in any part of the skin but has a particular predilection for the genital area. The skin lesions are papular and occur singly or in confluent patches. Extreme pallor of the tissues and a thin fragile epithelium with telangiectasia and gradual loss of the vulval contours may accompany the chronic phase, with the tissues becoming parchment-like. In early lesions bullae may form due to liquefaction and degeneration of the basal layer of the epithelium and dermal oedema. In childhood, rupture of these bullae may give a false impression of sexual abuse. Histologically, the epidermis is flat and thin but hyperkeratotic: there is striking hyalinisation of the upper dermis and a non-specific chronic inflammatory cell infiltrate of the lower dermis

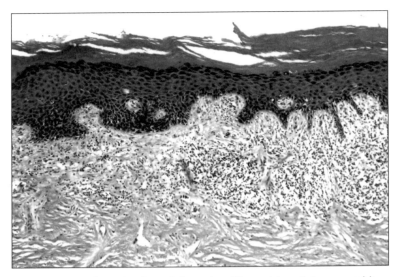

Figure 1.1 Lichen simplex of the vulva. The epidermis is covered by a thick layer of keratin and the epithelium is mildly thickened. The underlying stroma is infiltrated by chronic inflammatory cells.

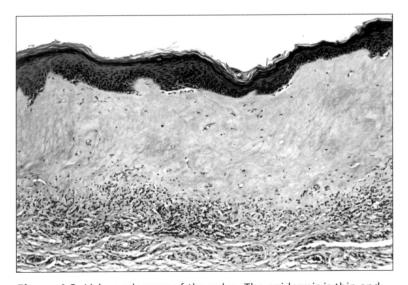

Figure 1.2 Lichen sclerosus of the vulva. The epidermis is thin and there is loss of the rete ridges. The superficial part of the underlying dermis is hyalinised whereas its deeper layers are infiltrated by lymphocytes.

(Figure 1.2). Lichen sclerosus may show secondary lichenification, this combination being previously classed as a 'mixed dystrophy'. Lichen sclerosus is not uncommonly found in association with vulvar squamous carcinoma but the magnitude of this risk has not been defined.

Inflammation of the vulva

NON-INFECTIVE VULVITIS

Non-infective inflammation of the vulva may be evoked by irritants, such as soap, scents, or deodorants. Excessive washing, especially if combined with the liberal use of antiseptics, may aggravate rather than alleviate the inflammation. Incontinence of urine, a copious vaginal discharge or excessive sweating can all be irritant to vulvar skin and severe vulvitis may follow exposure to radiotherapy.

INFECTIVE VULVITIS

Herpes virus infection

Herpetic vulvitis is not uncommon. It is acquired through sexual contact and occurs particularly in young women. The initial lesions are vesicular and usually painless. Later, the patient presents with a painful ulcerative vulvitis. The histological features of the infection tend to be non-specific and diagnosis is dependent upon serological studies or viral culture. Some women infected by the virus develop no signs or symptoms and can transmit the disease in the absence of clinical signs.

Human papillomavirus (HPV)

This results in the development of condylomata and vulvar intra-epithelial neoplasia (VIN) (see pages 4 and 6).

Granuloma inguinale

This disease, possibly sexually transmitted, is due to infection with the Gram-negative organism *Calymmatobacterium granulomatis* and is largely encountered in tropical countries. Primary lesions occur in the vulva as painful papules or nodules which break down to form a spreading ulcer with exuberant granulation tissue in its base. Healing of the lesions is by dense fibrosis which leads to extensive scarring: this may cause lymphatic obstruction with resultant brawny vulvar oedema. Histologically, there is a luxurious production of non-specific granulation tissue with an infiltrate of plasma cells and histiocytes: the latter contain the rounded or rod-like Donovan bodies which are diagnostic of this disease.

Lymphogranuloma venereum

This is a venereal infection with *Chlamydia trachomatis* and is most prevalent in the tropics and sub-tropics. The primary lesion is a self-healing vulvar papule or shallow ulcer which is later followed by a suppurative inguinal lymphadenitis: the large painful nodes become matted together and liquefy to form fluctuant buboes which drain through the skin via indolent sinuses. In a proportion of cases the primary lesions do not heal and progress to a chronic spreading destructive ulceration which may involve the vulva, vagina and rectum, leading eventually to vaginal and rectal stenoses. Histologically, characteristic features are present only in the lymph nodes where stellate abscesses are seen.

Syphilis

The vulva is a site of predilection for the primary lesion of syphilis, the chancre, which appears as a painless, hard, brownish-red nodule, often with surface erosion. This heals spontaneously after a few weeks. The typical silvery-grey snail-track ulcers of the secondary stage of syphilis can occur on the vulva, whereas elevated moist plaques, known as condylomata lata, may involve not only the vulva in secondary syphilis but also the adjacent perineum, perianal region and upper thighs.

Chancroid

This is a sexually-transmitted acute infection by *Haemophilus ducrei*. The primary lesions develop on the labia as painful nodules, often multiple, which break down to form small erosions. These tend to coalesce to form large ragged irregular ulcers with an excavated margin. The infection commonly spreads to the inguinal nodes to produce a painful lymphadenitis which may evolve into fluctuant masses that discharge through the skin. The histological appearances are of non-specific granulation tissue.

CONDYLOMA ACUMINATUM

These lesions, also known as venereal or genital warts, occur most commonly in young women and their incidence has been increasing in recent years. The condylomata typically occur along the edges of the labia minora, between the labia minora and majora, around the introitus and on the perineal and perianal skin. They are usually multiple and often confluent. Macroscopically, they appear as papillary or verrucous lesions which may be pedunculated or sessile. Histologically (Figure 1.3), complex fibrovascular cores are covered by acanthotic squamous epithelium which shows parakeratosis and, often, hyperkeratosis. Multinucleation, premature individual cell keratinisa-

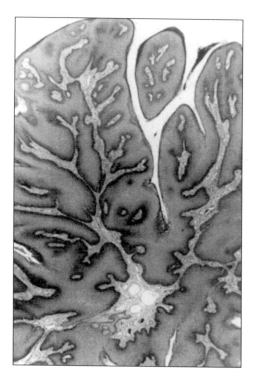

Figure 1.3 A condyloma acuminatum. Fine fibrovascular cores are covered by acanthotic epithelium which is mildly hyperkeratotic.

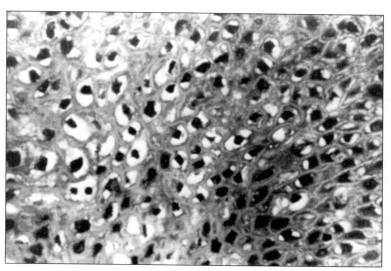

Figure 1.4 The epithelium in a condyloma. Numerous koilocytes are present.

tion and koilocytosis (Figure 1.4) are usually present.

Condylomata acuminata are due to infection with human papillomavirus (HPV) strains 6 or 11: the infection is usually sexually transmitted but is occasionally acquired in children as a result of non-sexual contact. They do not show any tendency to undergo neoplastic change but are, nevertheless, associated with an increased incidence of concomitant vulvar and cervical intraepithelial neoplasia (CIN).

Sometimes vulvar skin which appears normal to naked-eye examination may have histological features similar to those seen in the epithelium covering a condyloma acuminatum. Such lesions are called flat condylomata, or subclinical HPV infection, and have their counterparts on the cervix. Their significance lies in the fact that they, too, may be associated with VIN but may escape detection during ordinary clinical examination.

Non-invasive, intraepithelial neoplastic lesions

VIN

The term VIN encompasses and replaces those conditions previously known as Bowen's disease, Bowenoid papulosis, erythroplasia of Queyrat, squamous carcinoma *in situ* and dystrophy with atypia.

The incidence of VIN appears to have increased markedly during the last 25 years, particularly in younger women. In view of the high incidence of associated CIN, it is not surprising that many of the epidemiological factors operative for CIN, such as early onset of sexual activity, oral contraceptive use and multiple sexual partners, are also associated with VIN.

A clear association between VIN and HPV strain 16 infection has been abundantly demonstrated. A significant proportion of cases of VIN are, however, negative for HPV and it is now clear that there are two types of VIN. One, associated with HPV infection, occurs predominantly, but by no means solely, in younger patients and tends to be a multicentric and multifocal disease whilst the second, which is non-HPV-associated, is usually found in older women and is commonly unifocal and unicentric. There also appears to be a clear correlation between VIN and cigarette smoking in younger women.

The commonest complaint of women with VIN Stage 3 (see following page) is pruritus, but about one-third will have noticed an abnormality of the vulvar skin and a substantial proportion are asymptomatic, the lesion being detected incidentally during the investigation or treatment of a patient with vulvar condylomata, CIN, or abnormal cervical cytology by means of colposcopy, which should always include colposcopic evaluation of the vagina and vulva.

VIN may be discrete and sharply localised but can involve the entire vulva; the most frequent site for a discrete lesion is the labium minus.

The gross appearances are extremely variable for the lesions may be white, dull grey, red, brown, variegated red and white, or darkly pigmented and they may be flat, granular or warty.

Histologically, VIN may be undifferentiated or differentiated, the former tending to occur in younger women and being frequently associated with both HPV infection and smoking and the latter occurring more commonly in older women and often not associated with HPV infection.

The two basic patterns of undifferentiated VIN
- In basaloid VIN (Figure 1.5) cells of basal or parabasal type extend into the upper layers of the epidermis.
- In Bowenoid VIN (Figure 1.6) premature cellular maturation occurs, often in association with epithelial multinucleation, corps ronds and koilocytosis.

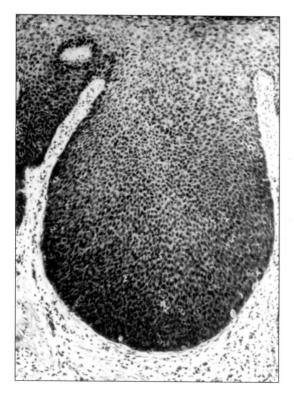

Figure 1.5 Basaloid type of VIN 3. The epithelium is occupied throughout its depth by cells resembling those of the normal basal layer.

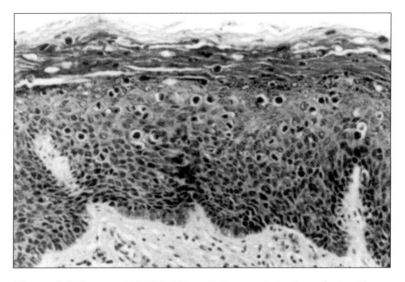

Figure 1.6 Bowenoid VIN 3. The cellular atypia is characterised by the presence of koilocytes, corps ronds and frequent mitoses.

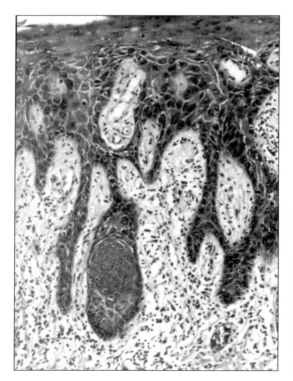

Figure 1.7 Differentiated VIN. Within the epithelium there is relatively little basal cellular atypia but there is a well-formed epithelial squamous pearl within an elongated rete ridge.

Common to both forms are the presence of often abnormal mitotic figures, above the basal layers of the epithelium, cellular and nuclear pleomorphism, a high nucleocytoplasmic ratio, irregular clumping of nuclear chromatin and, in many cases, either parakeratosis or hyperkeratosis. It is not uncommon in both forms of VIN for pigmentary incontinence to occur and for the underlying dermis to contain large numbers of melanin-laden macrophages, these being responsible for the pigmentation which is sometimes macroscopically apparent. The two forms of undifferentiated VIN may exist together in the same patient and are not mutually exclusive.

A differentiated VIN is one in which the epithelium shows little or no atypia above the basal or parabasal layers but large eosinophilic keratinocytes with abnormal nuclei are present in the basal layers and such cells, or intraepithelial pearls, are also present in the rete ridges (Figure 1.7).

It is usual to grade undifferentiated VIN, though the validity of such grading is open to debate.

- A lesion is classed as VIN 1 when cellular abnormalities and lack of both stratification and cytoplasmic differentiation are limited to the lower third of the epithelium.
- A lesion is classed as VIN 2 where extension of the abnormal cells into the middle third of the epithelium has occurred.
- A lesion is classed as VIN 3 when extension of abnormal cells into the upper third of the epithelium has occurred.

Grading of a basaloid VIN is relatively easy but the grading of a Bowenoid VIN is often difficult and sometimes impossible. A differentiated VIN cannot be graded but should probably be regarded, for clinical purposes, as a VIN 3.

Virtually nothing is known about the natural history of VIN 1 and 2 and the risk of such lesions evolving into an invasive carcinoma has not been determined; however, the risk is almost certainly very low.

There is no doubt that VIN 3 can progress to an invasive squamous cell carcinoma. Nevertheless, the potential for progression of VIN 3 to an invasive carcinoma, particularly the Bowenoid type in the younger patients, has generally been thought to be low and usually estimated to be no more than three to four percent. The risk of invasion is not, however, consistently low and it is possible that it has been seriously underestimated in the past, particularly in elderly women in whom progression to an invasive lesion can occur in up to 19% of VIN cases.

PAGET'S DISEASE

Vulvar Paget's disease is rare and occurs most commonly in post-menopausal women in whom it presents as often multiple, poorly – demarcated, erythematous areas in any part of the vulvar skin. Histologically (Figure 1.8), there are large, round or oval cells with pale cytoplasm, lying singly or in nests within the epidermis: glandular differentiation is seen in a few cases. The Paget cells contain mucus and are periodic acid-Schiff-positive after diastase digestion, characteristics which help to differentiate them from melanocytes.

Paget's disease of the vulva can arise in two ways. In a minority of cases there is a subjacent adnexal adenocarcinoma, the Paget cells representing an extension or metastasis from this to the epidermis. In most patients, however, there is no associated adenocarcinoma and the Paget cells develop *in situ* from pluripotential undifferentiated cells in the basal layers of the vulvar epithelium. Under these circumstances, the Paget cells represent an intraepithelial adenocarcinoma, which can occasionally progress to an invasive lesion.

Non-neoplastic cysts

Cysts forming in developmental remnants are those of mesonephric duct or peritoneal origin. The former develop in the lateral part of the labium majus and are lined by a cuboidal epithelium; they contain

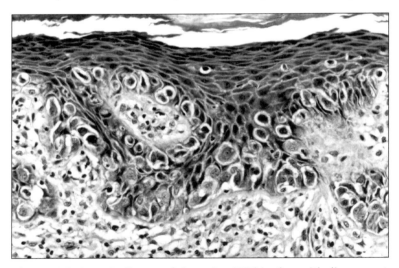

Figure 1.8 Paget's disease of the vulva. Within the epithelium, most markedly in the basal layers, there are groups of large Paget cells with pale cytoplasm.

clear serous fluid. Cysts of peritoneal origin develop in the fragment of peritoneum which may accompany the round ligament into the vulva; the resulting cyst is lined by mesothelium, contains clear watery fluid, and lies in the upper part of the labium majus.

Epidermoid cysts, which are lined by stratified squamous epithelium and contain laminated keratinous debris, occur most commonly in the labia majora, where they probably develop in the ducts of sebaceous glands, and in the perineal area where they occur in obstetric scars.

Obstruction of one of the minor mucus-secreting glands in the vestibule leads to the formation of a mucous cyst lined by a cubocolumnar, mucin-secreting epithelium. The largest and only individually named gland of this type is Bartholin's gland. Cysts developing in the gland duct lie in the posterolateral part of the labium majus and most commonly follow obstruction due to post-inflammatory fibrosis or inspissation of secretions. The cysts are lined by squamous, transitional or columnar epithelium (Figure 1.9), depending upon the level at which the obstruction occurred.

Benign tumours

Benign epithelial tumours of the vulva are more common than benign mesenchymal neoplasms, which are rare.

Epithelial tumours develop from the epidermis and the skin

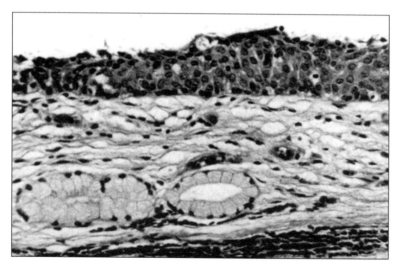

Figure 1.9 A cyst of Bartholin's gland duct. The cyst is lined (above) by transitional-type epithelium and within the wall there are secretory acini.

appendages. The most common of the epidermal tumours are the squamous papilloma, the fibroepitheliomatous polyp, basal cell papilloma and keratoacanthoma; occasionally intradermal or compound naevi are seen. Squamous papillomas and fibroepitheliomatous polyps (skin tags) are of similar appearance and consist of vascular connective tissue covered by mildly acanthotic and hyperkeratotic squamous epithelium; they are most common in the middle aged and elderly.

Basal cell papillomas (seborrhoeic keratoses) are small, exophytic, pigmented lesions which appear to be stuck on the skin. They are composed of sheets of small, regular cells resembling the normal basal cells of the epidermis and in many there are keratin-containing cysts.

Keratoacanthomas are rapidly-growing, self-limiting neoplasms which may be of viral origin. They consist of lobules of well-differentiated squamous cell masses arranged around a central keratin-plugged crater. Tumours may also develop from the sweat glands, one of the commonest of these in the vulva being the papillary hidradenoma. Hidradenomas are small, painless subcutaneous swellings, usually on the labia majora, and have a complex tubular, acinar and papillary histological pattern (Figure 1.10).

Vulval mesenchymal tumours have a tendency to become pedunculated. Fibromas, leiomyomas, lipomas, haemangiomas, neurofibromas, neurilemmomas and granular cell tumours occur.

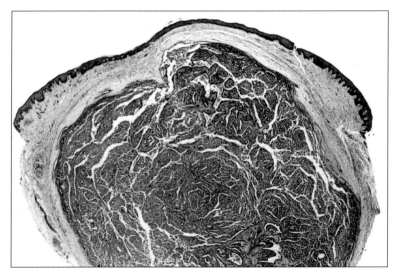

Figure 1.10 A hidradenoma of the vulva. Within the dermis there is a well-circumscribed nodule composed of tightly-packed glandular acini.

Malignant tumours

INVASIVE SQUAMOUS CELL CARCINOMA

Squamous cell carcinoma accounts for between 80 and 90% of malignant vulvar neoplasms and for about three to four percent of gynaecological cancers. Three-quarters of women with vulvar squamous cell carcinoma are aged over 60 years, the mean age at initial diagnosis being 66 years. The common presenting complaints are of a vulvar lump, pruritus, discharge, bleeding and pain.

The majority of squamous carcinomas (70%) develop on the labia, most commonly the labia majora; the second most common site is the clitoris. Over 50% of the tumours are ulcerated whilst about one-third are papillary and about ten percent are plaque-like.

Within recent years, squamous cell carcinomas of the vulva have been subdivided into three separate categories which differ from each other not only in their histological appearances but also in their relationship to patient age, association with HPV infection and origin from pre-existing VIN. These three categories are:
1   Typical keratinising squamous cell carcinoma.
2   Basaloid carcinoma.
3   Warty carcinoma.

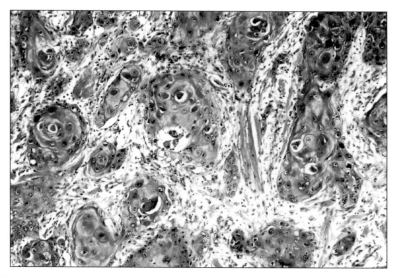

Figure 1.11 A well-differentiated keratinising squamous cell carcinoma of the vulva.

Typical keratinising squamous cell carcinomas (Figure 1.11) account for about 65% of cases, occur predominantly in women aged more than 65 years and are infrequently associated with HPV infection. The adjacent non-involved epithelium usually shows squamous hyperplasia or lichen sclerosus and VIN is relatively rarely seen. When present it tends to be of the differentiated type. Most are well-differentiated squamous cell carcinomas and form rounded nests of mature squamous cells with keratin pearls, with tongues of cells extending down into the dermis and subcutaneous tissues.

Basaloid carcinomas form about 28% of invasive neoplasms, are frequently associated with HPV strains 16 and 18 and occur in relatively young patients, usually below the age of 60 years. The adjacent non-involved epithelium commonly shows a basaloid type of VIN 3. The tumours are formed of masses, nests, clusters, or cords of basal-type cells with scanty cytoplasm and a high nucleo-cytoplasmic ratio.

Warty carcinomas constitute approximately 7% of invasive carcinomas, occur in younger patients and are associated with HPV strains 16 or 18 infection: the adjacent uninvolved epithelium usually shows a Bowenoid VIN 3. These tumours are formed of irregularly-shaped nests of epithelium in which there is a variable degree of nuclear pleomorphism and cytological atypia with multinucleated cells and koilocytes (Figure 1.12).

Squamous carcinomas spread directly to adjacent tissues, by the lymphatics to the inguinal, femoral and pelvic nodes and, rarely, late in

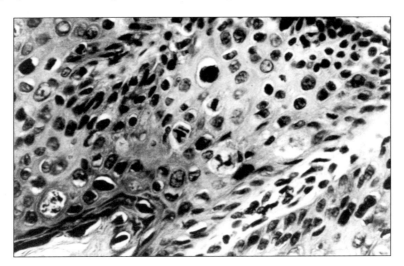

Figure 1.12 A Bowenoid carcinoma of the vulva which contains many koilocytes.

Table 1.1 Combined clinical and pathological staging of vulvar carcinoma (FIGO 1995)

Stage I	Tumour confined to the vulva, 2 cm or less in diameter, no metastases in the groin nodes Stage Ia depth of invasion not exceeding 1 mm (calculated from the nearest dermal papilla) Stage Ib all others
Stage II	Tumour confined to the vulva, more than 2 cm in diameter, no metastases in the groin nodes
Stage III	Tumour of any size with adjacent spread to the vagina, urethra and/or perineum and/or anus and/or unilateral pathologically-confirmed groin lymph node metastases
Stage IVa	Tumour of any size infiltrating the bladder mucosa and/or rectal mucosa, including the upper part of the urethral mucosa, and/or fixed to the bone and/or pathologically-confirmed bilateral groin lymph node metastases
Stage IVb	Distant metastases and/or pathologically-confirmed pelvic lymph node metastases

the course of the disease, by the bloodstream to the lungs, liver and bones. Nearly 30% of patients have inguinal nodal metastases at the time of initial diagnosis and 10–20% have pelvic node metastases.

The FIGO clinical staging system that was in use until relatively recently was highly inaccurate, particularly with respect to the presence or absence of groin lymph node metastases, and has now been replaced by a combined clinical and surgical staging system (Table 1.1). It is now accepted that that the presence of groin nodal metastases must be pathologically confirmed. The overall five-year survival rate for patients with vulvar carcinoma is now about 75%. For patients with no nodal metastases the survival rate is between 90 and 100% while for those with inguinal spread the survival rate is between 30 and 70%, falling to less than 25% if pelvic nodes are involved. The most important factor governing prognosis is the absence or otherwise of nodal spread and while various tumour-associated factors, such as tumour diameter, tumour thickness, tumour differentiation, tumour grade, the presence of vascular space invasion and pattern of tumour growth appear to be of prognostic value, it is probable that these are largely indicative of the risk of, and are subordinate to, nodal metastases.

VERRUCOUS CARCINOMA

This is a rare but distinctive variant of a squamous cell carcinoma. The tumour presents, usually in the postmenopausal years, as a slowly-growing, bulky, fungating, cauliflower-like mass. Histologically, these neoplasms have a remarkably bland appearance with little evidence of cellular atypia or mitotic activity. The base of the tumour is well circumscribed with bulbous rete ridges which appear to be compressing, rather than invading, the underlying tissues.

These tumours rarely metastasise to lymph nodes but tend to show a relentless local invasiveness and commonly recur after excision. Treatment is by surgery as they respond to radiotherapy by assuming an even more aggressive stance.

MALIGNANT MELANOMA

Between three and five percent of malignant melanomas in women occur in the vulvar skin. Such neoplasms constitute between four and five percent of all malignant vulvar tumours and occur predominantly in the sixth decade of life. The labia majora, labia minora and clitoris are involved with about equal frequency and the melanoma may be of the superficial spreading, nodular or acral lentiginous type.

The overall five-year survival rate for patients with a malignant melanoma of the vulva is about 30–40%, the tumour tending to spread early to the inguinal nodes and to be widely disseminated via the bloodstream. The prognosis for tumours still localised to the vulva depends upon the thickness of the neoplasm and its depth of invasion.

BASAL CELL CARCINOMA

Basal cell carcinomas account for only between two and ten percent of vulvar neoplasms and tend to develop on the labia majora in the elderly.

The tumours often present as a polypoidal or plaque-like ulcerated mass. The vulvar tumours are of a similar histological pattern and clinical behaviour to those encountered elsewhere in the body. About one-fifth recur locally after excision but lymph node metastases are exceptional.

MALIGNANT ADNEXAL (SKIN APPENDAGE) NEOPLASMS

These rare tumours present a wide variety of histological patterns and develop from sweat glands and sebaceous glands. Adenocarcinomas of tubular, myxoid and spindle cell form, apocrine adenocarcinomas resembling breast carcinoma, adenosquamous carcinomas, mucoid carcinomas and sebaceous carcinomas are all recognised. Local recurrence and metastasis are common.

CARCINOMA OF BARTHOLIN'S GLAND

Carcinomas of Bartholin's gland are rare and tend to occur at a peak age of about 50 years. The tumour usually presents as a vulvar nodule or mass which tends eventually to ulcerate through the overlying skin. Most of the neoplasms are either adenocarcinomas or squamous cell carcinomas (the latter probably arising from foci of metaplastic squamous epithelium within the ducts) but about 15% are adenoid cystic carcinomas.

Adenocarcinomas and squamous cell carcinomas tend to avail themselves of the rich lymphatic drainage of Bartholin's gland and metastasise first to the inguinal nodes then to the deep pelvic nodes, the five-year survival rate for patients with these tumours being only about 30%. Adenoid cystic adenocarcinomas show less tendency to metastasise but are locally highly aggressive, invading extensively and recurring with considerable frequency.

URETHRAL CARCINOMA

Urethral carcinoma, although rare, is more common in women than men, affecting particularly old or elderly women. Tumours of the distal urethra are more common than those in the proximal, or posterior, urethra.

In the distal urethra, tumours are usually squamous or transitional, whereas in the proximal urethra adenocarcinomas also occur. Patients in whom disease is limited to the distal urethra do well but tumours involving the whole urethra or only its proximal portion have a poor prognosis because in many such cases metastases have already occurred at the time of diagnosis.

METASTATIC TUMOURS

The possibility that rare tumours of the vulva, such as adenocarcinoma, might be metastases should always be borne in mind, as the vulva is not an uncommon site of metastases from the cervix, endometrium, vagina, ovary, urethra, kidney, breast, rectum and lung.

2 The vagina

Vaginal inflammation

NON-INFECTIVE INFLAMMATION

Non-infective vaginal inflammation may complicate trauma, surgery, irradiation, the introduction of foreign bodies, the application of chemical substances, or the wearing of a pessary. These factors are more likely to cause inflammatory changes at times of oestrogen deficiency, for example after the menopause.

INFECTIVE INFLAMMATION

Most vaginal infections are sexually transmitted but it is far from certain how the infecting organisms become established in the vagina and overcome the dual threats posed by the normal vaginal flora and the acidity of vaginal fluids. It is probable that changes in oestrogen or progesterone levels are an important factor in the establishment of an infection in so far as oestrogen deficiency or progesterone excess will result in diminished epithelial growth, a reduction in the supply of glycogen and restriction of the ability of lactobacilli to flourish, thus allowing invading organisms to gain an ascendancy.

Bacterial vaginosis

The sexually-transmitted Gram-negative bacillus, *Gardnerella vaginalis,* either acting singly or in combination with anaerobic organisms, is now recognised to be the cause of the vast majority of cases previously designated as 'non-specific vaginitis'. Bacterial vaginosis is associated with a thin, watery, highly malodorous vaginal discharge but the organism is only a surface parasite and does not invade the vaginal tissues or evoke any inflammatory reaction.

Candidiasis

Candida albicans may exist in the vagina without causing any signs or symptoms. The fungal organism can, however, change from a saprophyte to a pathogen if the host is immunosuppressed or if growth of the normal vaginal flora is inhibited by, for example, the use of broad-spectrum antibiotics. Such a change also often occurs in pregnancy when high oestrogen levels may be associated with increased cellular glycogen concentration. Once allowed to proliferate freely, *C. albicans* penetrates focally into the vaginal epithelium and initiates a vaginitis. The vaginal epithelium is congested and whitish plaques may be seen on the vaginal surface; these are easily removed to expose a reddened 'raw' area.

Trichomoniasis

The unicellular protozoal parasite *Trichomonas vaginalis* is one of the commonest causes of a vaginitis. The parasite is usually sexually transmitted but can on occasion be transmitted via fomites. The acute stage of the infection is characterised by a frothy vaginal discharge and the vaginal skin has a reddish granular appearance. Histologically, congestion, oedema, and a lymphoplasmocytic infiltrate of the subepithelial papillae are characteristic features. The inflammatory infiltrate may extend into the epithelium and form small intraepithelial abscesses. The infection may progress into a chronic state, although some women become symptomless carriers of the parasite.

Gonorrhoea

The thick squamous epithelium of the adult vagina is resistant to gonococcal infection. In children, however, the thin epithelium is permeable to the organism, which can produce a vaginitis.

Syphilis

The vagina is an uncommon site for a chancre but the mucosal 'snail-track' ulcers and condylomata lata of secondary syphilis occur with some frequency in the lower vagina. Tertiary-stage lesions are only rarely encountered in the vagina.

Vaginal adenosis

This condition, which is usually asymptomatic but is occasionally associated with a vaginal discharge, is characterised by the presence of glandular structures in the lamina propria of the vagina (Figure 2.1), with some opening on to the vaginal surface. The glands are most commonly lined by a mucinous, endocervical-type epithelium but may have a lining of endometrial or tubal type. The glands have a marked tendency to undergo squamous metaplasia, and in older women may eventually be completely replaced by squamous tissue.

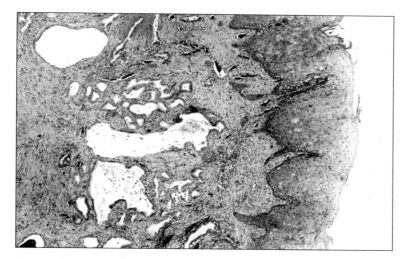

Figure 2.1 Vaginal adenosis. The vagina is lined by stratified squamous epithelium and the underlying stroma contains a series of glands, some lined by a mucus-secreting epithelium and others by endometrial-type epithelium.

Vaginal adenosis is thought to be due to sequestration of Müllerian elements during vaginal embryogenesis and is indicative of a disturbance in the orderly replacement of the lower parts of the Müllerian ducts by the squamous epithelium of the urogenital sinus. The condition may occur spontaneously but is particularly common in girls who have been exposed prenatally to diethylstilboestrol (DES), being found in 70% of girls exposed to DES during the first eight weeks of fetal life.

Vaginal adenosis is not, in itself, of any major clinical importance but is of considerable significance as a precursor of the clear-cell adenocarcinoma of the vagina (see below).

Vaginal intraepithelial neoplasia (VAIN)

VAIN has been studied much less intensively than have vulvar (VIN) and cervical (CIN) intraepithelial neoplasia and its natural history is poorly understood. The lesion is often multifocal, usually asymptomatic and is discovered only on routine examination, when it is seen either as an area of increased vascularity or as a whitish patch. A high proportion of women with VAIN have been previously treated for either intraepithelial or invasive neoplasia of the cervix and it is thought that the aetiological factors for VAIN are similar to those for CIN (see page 33).

The histological appearances of VAIN are similar to those of both VIN and CIN and include delayed maturation of the squamous cells, disturbance in polarity, an increased nucleo-cytoplasmic ratio, nuclear pleomorphism, the finding of mitotic figures above the basal layers, and the presence of abnormal mitotic figures.

- A lesion is classed as VAIN 1 when undifferentiated cells are confined to the lower third of the epithelium.
- A lesion is classed as VAIN 2 when undifferentiated cells extend into the middle third of the epithelium.
- A lesion is classed as VAIN 3 when differentiated cells either extend into the upper third of the epithelium or occupy its full thickness.

VAIN is widely regarded as a precursor of an invasive squamous cell carcinoma of the vagina but neither its invasive potential nor its quantitative importance as a precursor of a malignant vaginal neoplasm have been adequately defined.

Vaginal neoplasms

Malignant neoplasms of the vagina are rare, accounting for only about one percent of cancers of the female genital tract. A malignant neoplasm in the vagina is more likely to be a metastasis from sites such as the colon, endometrium or kidney than a primary vaginal tumour.

SQUAMOUS CARCINOMA

Neoplasms of this type account for 95% of malignant vaginal tumours and occur predominantly in women in their sixth or seventh decades. Squamous carcinomas develop most commonly in the posterior wall of the upper third of the vagina, usually present as an exophytic fungating mass and are often moderately well differentiated. The tumour invades, at a relatively early stage, adjacent structures such as the cervix, prevaginal tissues, bladder and rectum. Lymphatic spread from tumours in the upper vagina is to the iliac and obturator nodes, whereas that from neoplasms in the lower vagina is to the femoral and inguinal nodes. The current overall five-year survival rate is about 30%.

The aetiology of vaginal squamous carcinoma is unknown but it has been suggested that long-standing procidentia or the prolonged wearing of a pessary may be of some aetiological importance. This may well be true, but these factors are of little importance in current practice. The role of HPV infection in the aetiology of vaginal carcinoma is currently undetermined.

CLEAR-CELL ADENOCARCINOMA

Vaginal neoplasms of this type used to be of extreme rarity but their incidence has increased in recent years, this increase being entirely in young girls who have been exposed prenatally to DES. Approximately one in 1500 women exposed to DES during the first 18 weeks of their prenatal life will develop a clear-cell adenocarcinoma, the tumour usually becoming apparent between the ages of 14 and 23 years, most commonly in girls aged 17–19 years. The tumour almost certainly originates in pre-existing vaginal adenosis and is therefore of Müllerian origin.

A clear-cell adenocarcinoma usually develops in the upper third of the vagina and may form a polypoid, nodular, or papillary mass. Histologically (Figure 2.2), there is a complex mixture of solid papillary, tubular and cystic patterns, the solid areas being formed by sheets of cells with clear cytoplasm and the tubules being lined by 'hobnail' cells which have large nuclei that protrude into the tubular lumen.

The tumour spreads by local invasion, the lymphatics and the bloodstream. Although the pelvic nodes are commonly the site of metastases, there is a surprisingly high incidence of spread to the supraclavicular nodes. Blood-borne dissemination is principally to the lungs. Treatment is by radical surgery and the overall five-year survival rate is 80%.

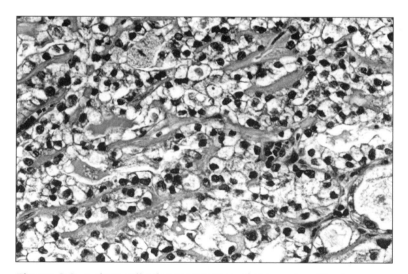

Figure 2.2 A clear-cell adenocarcinoma of the vagina. The tumour is composed of large cells with well-defined cell margins and clear cytoplasm.

SARCOMA BOTRYOIDES

This term is applied to the rare embyronal rhabdomyosarcoma of the vagina, a tumour which most commonly occurs in the first five years of life. The neoplasm arises from the connective tissues of the vaginal wall and tends to form a polypoid mass of greyish-red haemorrhagic tissue which may fill and protrude from the vagina. Histologically, there is typically a widely dispersed population of pleomorphic immature mesenchymal cells, rhabdomyoblasts and striated muscle cells set in an abundant oedematous or myxoid stroma. The epithelium covering the tumour is bland and the neoplastic cells tend to be condensed below this to form a 'cambium' layer. A vaginal sarcoma botryoides infiltrates locally into the pelvic tissues and has a poor prognosis.

3 The cervix

Physiological changes in the cervix

ECTOPY OR ECTROPION

In the pre-pubertal girl the squamo-columnar junction lies around the external os or on the ectocervix. At the time of puberty, in pregnancy (particularly the first one) and in many steroid contraceptive users, changes in the hormonal milieu result in an alteration in the shape and an increase in the bulk of the cervix. This results in eversion of the endocervical epithelium with the squamo-columnar junction being carried passively further out on to the anatomical ectocervix. This rim of endocervical tissue forms an ectopy or ectropion exposed around the external os. The ectopy appears red through the thin covering epithelium and the surface is villous.

The exposure of the delicate endocervical epithelium to the acid environment of the vagina leads to squamous metaplasia with the squamous epithelial cells differentiating from pluripotential uncommitted cells. Squamous metaplasia is a protective mechanism in which relatively fragile endocervical columnar epithelium is replaced by a more robust squamous epithelium.

The metaplastic squamous epithelium occludes the mouths of the endocervical crypts with the resultant formation of retention cysts or Nabothian follicles. This process also restores the position of the squamo-columnar junction to the external os. The area of squamous metaplasia is termed the transformation zone and is the site at which the majority of cervical neoplasms arise. In young women the transformation zone lies where it develops, on the ectocervix, but after the age of 30 years there is an increasing tendency, because of shrinkage of the soft tissue of the cervix, for the squamo-columnar junction to be retracted and come to lie within the endocervical canal; hence that area of epithelium which formed the transformation zone is also withdrawn to within the canal. An endocervical squamo-columnar junction is a virtually constant finding after the menopause.

PREGNANCY

In pregnancy, in addition to the development of an ectopy, there is a spongy enlargement of the cervix because of congestion and oedema. Surface maturation of the squamous epithelium is absent because of progesterone predominance in the hormonal milieu. Focal decidualisation of the stroma is common. The columnar epithelium of the ectopy or endocervical canal often undergoes a form of hyperplasia to form tightly-packed glands or tubules lined by flattened or cuboidal cells. This condition of microglandular hyperplasia is, in most cases, only a microscopic change, though it may on rare occasions form polypoid nodules which bleed on touch.

Inflammatory disease of the cervix

Cervical inflammation (cervicitis) may occur as an isolated lesion or as part of a more widespread inflammatory process in the genital tract. The histological appearances are, however, remarkably stereotyped and often give no clue as to the aetiology (Figure 3.1). Inflammation may be acute, active chronic, or chronic and chronic inflammation may be granulomatous or non-granulomatous. There is a normal population of plasma cells and lymphocytes in the stroma adjacent to the external cervical os and these often lead to an unwarranted diag-

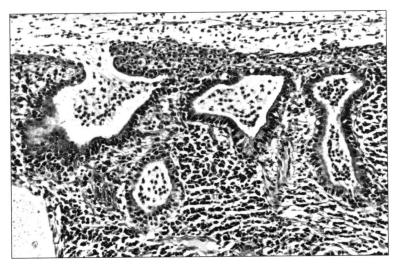

Figure 3.1 Severe cervical inflammation. The cervical crypts are distended by an acute inflammatory exudate, there is ulceration of the surface epithelium and the stroma is infiltrated by lymphocytes, plasma cells and macrophages.

nosis of cervicitis. Hence the recognition of an inflammatory process depends upon the presence not only of inflammatory cells but also upon the finding of associated changes such as a reduction in mucus secretion, infiltration of the epithelium by inflammatory cells, ulceration, the formation of granulation tissue, fibrosis, the development of lymphoid follicles with germinal centres or granuloma formation.

Acute inflammation is characterised by oedema and congestion, the presence in the stroma and crypts of polymorphonuclear leucocytes and by the outpouring of an acute inflammatory exudate. In severe cases there may be abscess formation and ulceration of the surface epithelium. In persistent or active chronic inflammation the infiltrate becomes plasma-lymphocytic and histiocytic with scanty polymorphonuclear leucocytes, whilst in some chronic infections lymphoid follicles or granulomas are a characteristic feature.

NON-INFECTIVE INFLAMMATION

Inflammation occurs following surgery, parturition, cryosurgery, laser therapy, cautery, the use of douches or ointments and in association with the wearing of an intrauterine contraceptive device (IUCD). The cervix often becomes inflamed if there is a prolapse, and this is particularly marked if ulceration occurs – this is due to a combination of tissue ischaemia following alterations in the blood supply to the cervix as it descends and rubbing from clothing and is termed decubital ulceration.

INFECTIVE INFLAMMATION

Many infections of the cervix are of a non-specific polymicrobial nature. Bacterial infections tend particularly to involve the endocervix or an ectopy, partly because the deep crypts afford a safe harbour to the organisms, partly because the columnar epithelium in these sites offers less resistance to infection than does the stratified squamous epithelium of the ectocervix and partly because organisms sequestrated in the cervical crypts may not be affected by either systemic or local therapeutic agents. Chronic cervical inflammation occurs particularly when there is obstruction to, and stasis of, cervical secretions and is therefore encountered when the vagina is obstructed by a foreign body or tumour or when the endocervical canal is blocked by a neoplasm, polyp, or stricture. The resultant scarring and fibrosis leads to further crypt destruction, thus increasing the obstruction and perpetuating the inflammatory process. The organisms most commonly isolated in such circumstances include coliforms, commensals, mycoplasma, *Gardnerella vaginalis,* and *Chlamydia,* but their role in initiating the inflammation is uncertain.

SPECIFIC INFECTIONS

Viral infections

HERPES SIMPLEX VIRUS TYPE 2

Herpetic infection of the cervix is most common in teenagers and young adults and is usually associated with infection of the vulva and vagina. Symptoms develop three to seven days after inoculation and are most severe in primary infections. Although healing is usually rapid and complete, recurrences are frequent and an asymptomatic infected state may develop.

Focal necrosis of the squamous epithelium of the cervix leads to the development of shallow ulcers and rarely to the development of a necrotising cervicitis or a chronic inflammatory mass which may be mistaken for a carcinoma.

HUMAN PAPILLOMAVIRUS (HPV)

Cervical infection by this sexually-transmitted organism is increasingly common. HPV infection can result in condylomata or flat 'warty' lesions and is also being increasingly regarded as being of aetiological importance in cervical neoplasia (see pages 31 and 32 [condylomata and neoplasia]).

Bacterial infection

NEISSERIA GONORRHOEAE

The squamous epithelium of the ectocervix is relatively resistant to infection by this highly-contagious organism. Gonococci can, however, pass through the columnar epithelium of the endocervix to elicit an acute exudative endocervicitis characterised by stromal congestion and oedema and a seropurulent exudate while the columnar epithelium becomes focally degenerate and ulcerated.

Infection may clear, become chronic, or spread to the endometrium and fallopian tubes. A proportion of patients become asymptomatic carriers, while others develop chronic gonococcal cervicitis with pericryptal fibrosis, crypt distortion and stasis of cervical secretions.

CHLAMYDIA INFECTION

Chlamydial infection of the cervix is characterised by the development of a follicular cervicitis (Figure 3.2).

The inflammatory infiltrate, which is often very heavy, is composed of plasma cells and lymphocytes which form lymphoid follicles with germinal centres. Intraepithelial abscesses and ulceration of the overlying epithelium may develop in severe cases.

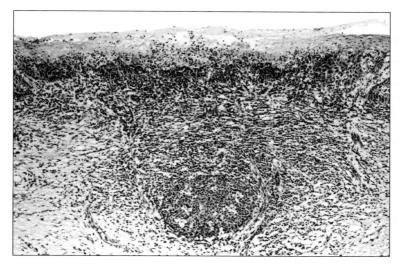

Figure 3.2 Follicular cervicitis. In addition to a diffuse chronic inflammatory cell infiltrate, there is a lymphoid follicle with a germinal centre. These appearances are highly suggestive of a chlamydial infection.

SPIROCHAETAL INFECTION

The primary lesion of syphilis occurs in the cervix in up to 40% of cases, where it may form a typical hard, ulcerated chancre. Occasionally multiple small ulcers form which resemble those seen in herpetic cervicitis, and, rarely, a fungating mass resembling a neoplasm may develop. When the chancre lies in the endocervix the entire cervix may become indurated and oedematous.

The characteristic histological findings are a dense, subepithelial plasma cell infiltrate, a perivascular infiltrate of lymphocytes with endothelial hyperplasia and, in long-standing cases, endarteritis. The mucous patches, but not the condylomata lata of the secondary stage of syphilis, may occur on the cervix but this is an exceptionally rare site for a gumma.

Protozoal and other infections

TRICHOMONAS VAGINALIS

Infection of the vagina and cervix by *T. vaginalis* are inseparable. The mucosa of the infected cervix is reddened and the underlying vessels are ectatic, appearing as red spots and leading to the descriptive term, a 'strawberry' cervix. The epithelium is infiltrated by polymorphonuclear leucocytes and is partly desquamated with the underlying stroma containing chronic inflammatory cells. In many cases the infection resolves following treatment but in others it may become chronic as the endocervical crypts act as a reservoir of infection.

SCHISTOSOMIASIS

Schistosomiasis of the cervix is rarely seen in the UK but it is a common genital tract pathogen in some areas of the world. Cervical infection leads to the development of a bulky indurated cervix or a polypoidal mass and there is a granulomatous response to the ova. Progressive fibrosis may cause gross cervical distortion.

Cervical polyps

These are common and arise in 95% of cases from the endocervix. An endocervical polyp represents a focal overgrowth of hyperplastic endocervical epithelium and its underlying stroma but the cause of this overgrowth is unknown.

The polyps form pedunculated, round or ovoid masses of pinkish tissue which grow into the endocervical canal. Histologically, they have a surface epithelium of columnar endocervical-type epithelium which forms crypt-like infoldings into the stroma of the polyp (Figure 3.3). Squamous metaplasia of the surface epithelium is common.

Endocervical polyps occur most frequently in women aged 30–50 years and there is no risk of malignant change.

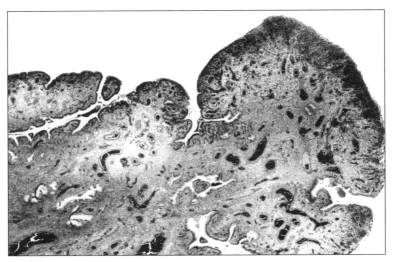

Figure 3.3 A cervical polyp. The polyp is composed of endocervical tissue containing congested blood vessels and is ulcerated at its apex.

Condylomata of the cervix

Cervical warts, or condyloma acuminata, have long been recognised but it is only in recent years that the flat condyloma (also known as 'warty atypia', 'condyloma planum' and 'non-condylomatous cervical wart virus infection') has been identified. Both lesions are due to a sexually-transmitted infection with HPV and it is now realised that flat condylomata account for over 90% of HPV infections of the cervix.

Condylomata acuminata are seen as fleshy, pointed papules which are often multiple and sometimes confluent. A flat condyloma is, by contrast, not visible to the naked eye and, although often suggested by an abnormal cervical smear, is detectable only on colposcopy and histology. Histologically, the hallmark of an HPV infection is the presence, within squamous epithelium, of koilocytes. These cells have enlarged, irregular, hyperchromatic nuclei with a prominent clear perinuclear space (halo) and margination of the cytoplasm.

Multinucleation and premature individual cell keratinisation (dyskeratosis) are other typical features of HPV infection.

Condylomata occur most commonly in the squamous epithelium of the transformation zone of young women and HPV strains 6, 11, 16, or 18 have been identified in a very high proportion of these lesions. Condylomata due to infection with HPV-6 or HPV-11 almost invariably pursue a benign course. Some regress spontaneously while the remainder may persist in the absence of treatment in an unchanged state for many years. Condylomata due to HPV strains 16 and 18 are, however, frequently complicated by a superimposed CIN and it should be noted that condylomata due to these strains of HPV are always of the flat variety.

Cervical neoplasms

Squamous carcinomas, adenocarcinomas and adenosquamous carcinomas all occur in the cervix but squamous tumours predominate to the extent that there is a tendency to think of cervical cancer only in terms of squamous carcinoma. This undoubtedly blurs our understanding of the aetiology, pathogenesis and development of the different tumours.

SQUAMOUS NEOPLASIA

Both pre-invasive and invasive squamous neoplasms occur. The condition of CIN is thought to represent an intraepithelial neoplasm and this term is used to encompass those abnormalities previously described as dysplasia and carcinoma *in situ*. This lesion occurs, in the vast majority of cases, in that area of metaplastic squamous epithelium which was the transformation zone. CIN may, therefore, develop on the anatomical ectocervix or within the endocervical canal and is a recognised precursor of invasive squamous carcinoma.

Invasive and intraepithelial squamous neoplasia of the cervix have, as might be expected, aetiological factors in common and it is therefore convenient to discuss the aetiology of both conditions together. Some adenocarcinomas and adenosquamous carcinomas appear to share common aetiological factors with squamous carcinomas but other adenocarcinomas have different aetiological correlates.

During the process of metaplasia, the immature squamous epithelium of the transformation zone appears to be particularly susceptible to oncogenic stimuli. Various factors have been identified which may be of aetiological importance in the development of pre-invasive and invasive neoplasia of the cervix, although final proof of their significance is still lacking. They can be divided into epidemiological factors and causative agents.

It is almost unknown for CIN or invasive squamous carcinoma of the cervix to develop in women who have never had coitus and the greater the number of sexual partners she or her consort have had and the younger her age at first coitus, the greater her risk of developing cervical carcinoma. There is a relatively high frequency of sexually-transmitted disease in women with cervical neoplasia but this may simply be related to the likelihood of a greater number of sexual partners. Patients with cervical carcinoma are more likely to come from the lower than the upper socio-economic groups which may reflect differences in sexual behaviour between these two groups.

There is a slightly increased risk of cervical neoplasia in women who use oral contraception and a decreased risk for those using a barrier form of contraception. The protection offered by barrier methods may reflect the fact that exposure of the cervix to seminal plasma results in local immunosuppression but may also indicate the ability of barrier contraception to prevent the transmission of an aetiological agent. Oral contraception allows the transmission of such an agent and also alters the hormonal milieu of the cervix.

Cigarette smoking is an independent risk factor for cervical neoplasia. This may be due to the excretion in the cervical mucus of chemicals derived from tobacco smoke which are not only capable of exerting a carcinogenic effect but also appear to cause local immunosuppression.

All the epidemiological data indicate that a sexually-transmitted agent is implicated in the aetiology of cervical neoplasia and there is now overwhelming evidence that a central role is played by certain strains of HPV, particularly strains 16 and 18. Infection with these viruses is common in young women but the vast majority of such infections are transient, with the virus being rapidly cleared from the cervix. The women at risk for cervical neoplasia are those in whom the viral infection persists. The reasons for viral persistence in a small proportion of women are unknown but co-factors such as smoking, local immunosuppression and other synergistic viral infections may be of importance.

It is probable that HPV is present in all cervical squamous cell carcinomas and is often integrated into the host genome. Some indication of how these viruses act as oncogenic agents has come from the demonstration that the proteins coded for by the E6 and E7 genes of HPV-16 or -18 combine with, and result in the degradation of, the tumour-suppressor gene p53.

CIN usually occurs at a younger age than does squamous carcinoma, which has its peak incidence in women over the age of 45 years. In recent years, although the incidence of carcinoma in women between the ages of 35 and 45 has declined, the incidence in women under the age of 35 has increased and there has been little change in incidence in women over the age of 45 years. There are still approximately 1500 deaths a year from cervical cancer in England and Wales and the incidence of CIN has shown a dramatic increase.

CIN

CIN is a single continuous disease process that is characterised histologically by a failure of the normal process of maturation in the squamous epithelium of the transformation zone together with a variable degree of nuclear enlargement and pleomorphism. In the UK, CIN is graded into CIN 1, CIN 2 and CIN 3 and this terminology is preferred to that of the Bethesda system which includes flat condylomata within its grading system and simply recognises two entities of 'high- and low-grade squamous intraepithelial lesions'.

- CIN 1 (Figure 3.4) is recognised by a lack of maturation of cells in the lower third of the squamous epithelium (though cytoplasmic maturation occurs in the upper two-thirds of the epithelium) together with mild nuclear atypia.
- In CIN 2 (Figure 3.5) there is a failure of the cells to mature in the lower one- to two-thirds of the epithelium and a greater degree of nuclear atypia.
- In CIN 3 (Figure 3.6) undifferentiated cells extend into the upper third of the epithelium or occupy its full thickness.

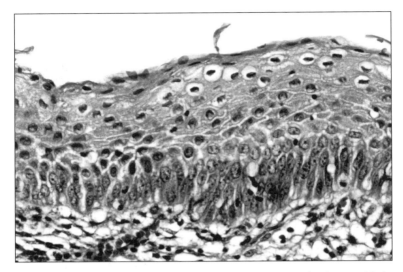

Figure 3.4 Cervical intraepithelial neoplasia, CIN 1. The lower third of the epithelium is occupied by cells with large nuclei and a high nucleo-cytoplasmic ratio: they lack differentiation.

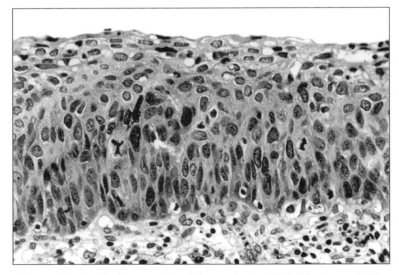

Figure 3.5 Cervical intraepithelial neoplasia, CIN 2. The lower half of the epithelium is occupied by cells lacking differentiation: a tripolar mitotic figure is present.

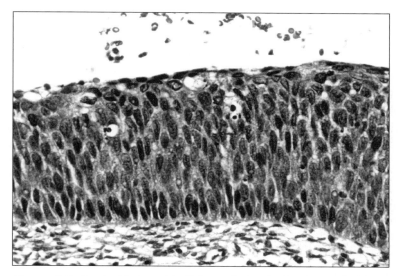

Figure 3.6 Cervical intraepithelial neoplasia, CIN 3. The epithelium is occupied throughout its full thickness by undifferentiated cells with large hyperchromatic nuclei and high nucleo-cytoplasmic ratios.

Features indicative of HPV infection are present in many cases, these being the presence of koilocytes, epithelial multinucleation and individual cell keratinisation. These abnormalities are most evident in CIN 1 and 2 and are least apparent in CIN 3. CIN 3 is usually assumed to be a squamous intraepithelial neoplasm but can be closely mimicked by a very poorly differentiated adenocarcinoma *in situ*, which can be recognised only by the use of a mucin stain.

The grade of CIN is rarely uniform throughout the affected area of the transformation zone. Generally it is of lower grade at the outer ectocervical margin, adjacent to the ectocervical squamous epithelium and of higher grade centrally.

In the transformation zone, metaplasia is not always limited to the surface epithelium and, similarly, CIN may also extend into the underlying endocervical crypts.

When invasion occurs from CIN, it may occur from the surface epithelium or from crypts and, although the epithelium from which invasion has occurred most commonly has the features of CIN 3, invasion may less commonly occur from CIN 1 or 2.

CIN is a precursor of invasive squamous cell carcinoma but not all, or even most, cases of CIN will progress to an invasive neoplasm. It is probable that approximately 35–40% of cases of CIN 3 will evolve into an invasive squamous cell carcinoma within 20 years of diagnosis if untreated. The long-term risk of invasive neoplasia in cases of CIN 1 and 2 is less well defined but in any individual patient either of these forms of CIN carries the risk of eventual squamous cell carcinoma.

MICROINVASIVE CARCINOMA (STAGE IA INVASIVE CARCINOMA)

Invasion from intraepithelial neoplasia is first recognised by an increase in the amount of cytoplasm and eosinophilia of the cytoplasm in one or more cells in the basal layer of the squamous epithelium covering the surface of the cervix or lining one or more of the crypts. Subsequently, the deep margin of the epithelium becomes irregular and jagged as tongues of infiltrating cells penetrate the underlying stroma (Figure 3.7) where they evoke a lymphocytic infiltrate and, sometimes, local stromal oedema or fibrosis.

Microinvasive carcinoma is the term used to describe a degree of invasion which is associated with minimal risk of nodal metastasis and is sufficiently small to treat in many cases by local or conservative means. It may be multifocal or limited to a single focus. It must not exceed 7mm in its greatest horizontal axis and must not penetrate the stroma for more than 5mm. With the smallest lesions, a minor degree of lymphatic permeation in the immediate vicinity of the neoplasm

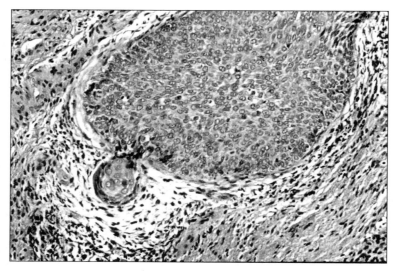

Figure 3.7 Microinvasive carcinoma of the cervix (Stage Ia1 invasive carcinoma). A tongue of squamous epithelium is invading the superficial stroma from a crypt which is lined by epithelium showing CIN 3.

does not exclude the lesion from this category. Earlier descriptions of microinvasive carcinoma in terms only of its depth of penetration are now regarded as having little value and can be misleading and potentially dangerous.

INVASIVE SQUAMOUS CELL CARCINOMA

Squamous carcinomas constitute about 70% of all malignant cervical neoplasms. They can occur at any age from 17 to 70 years but develop most commonly in women in their sixth decade.

Squamous carcinoma may develop either on the ectocervix, where it tends to grow in a predominantly exophytic manner to form a papillary or polypoidal mass, or in the endocervical canal where it commonly expands the cervix to form a hard barrel-shaped mass. Ulceration and necrosis are common features and the tumours often bleed on touch.

Histologically, squamous cell carcinoma infiltrates cervical stroma as a network of anastomosing bands which appear in cross-section as irregular islands with spiky or angular margins. The tumours may be well differentiated (the large-cell keratinising type) (Figure 3.8), moderately differentiated (large-cell focally keratinising type) or poorly differentiated (large- or small-cell non-keratinising types) (Figure 3.9). As 80% are either moderately or poorly differentiated tumours, well-differentiated neoplasms are the exception rather than the rule.

Squamous cell carcinomas spread locally to invade the uterine body, vagina, bladder and rectum with the spread occurring along the paracervical ligaments to the lateral side walls of the pelvis, surrounding and compressing the ureters as they traverse the paracervical region. Lymphatic spread is to the paracervical, iliac, obturator and para-aortic nodes but dissemination by this route does not occur methodically and an absence of metastases from the iliac nodes is no guarantee that tumour will not be present in para-aortic nodes. Blood-borne spread is a late phenomenon and is principally to the liver, lungs and skeleton.

Delineation of prognostic factors for patients with invasive cervical squamous carcinoma is probably only of real value in those with Stage Ib or IIa disease. In such cases the two most important factors governing the prognosis are the extent of the local disease and the presence or otherwise of nodal metastases. The extent of the local disease is usually defined by clinical examination (Table 3.1) but to a very significant extent the prognosis depends upon whether nodal metastases are present or not. Tumour differentiation is probably not of prognostic significance while factors such as tumour size and vascular space invasion are surrogates for the risk of nodal metastasis rather than independent prognostic indices.

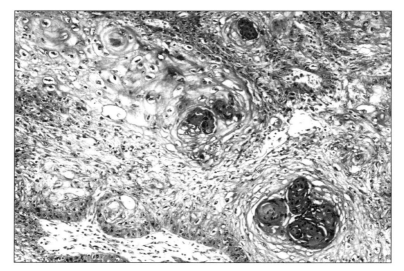

Figure 3.8 A well-differentiated keratinising squamous cell carcinoma of the cervix.

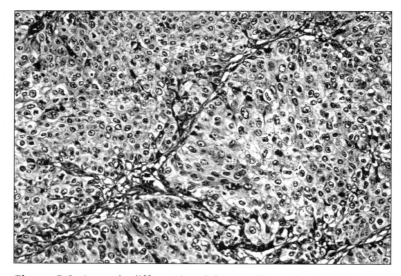

Figure 3.9 A poorly-differentiated, large cell, non-keratinising squamous cell carcinoma of the cervix.

Table 3.1 1995 modification of FIGO staging of carcinoma of the cervix

Stage 0	Preinvasive carcinoma (CIN 3, carcinoma in situ)
Stage I	Carcinoma confined to the cervix (extension of the corpus should be disregarded)
	Stage Ia measured stromal invasion with maximum depth of 5 mm and no wider than 7 mm
	Stage Ia1 measured invasion of stroma up to 3 mm in depth and no wider than 7 mm
	Stage Ia2 measured invasion of stroma 3–5 mm in depth and no wider than 7 mm
	Stage Ib Clinical lesions confined to the cervix or preclinical lesions greater than Stage Ia
	Stage Ib1 Clinical lesions no greater than 4 cm in size
	Stage Ib2 Clinical lesions greater than 4 cm in size
Stage II	Invasive carcinoma that extends beyond the cervix but has not reached either lateral pelvic wall: involvement of the vagina is limited to the upper two-thirds
Stage III	Invasive carcinoma that extends to either lateral pelvic wall and/or the lower third of the vagina
Stage IV	Invasive carcinoma that involves urinary bladder and/or rectum or extends beyond the true pelvis

GLANDULAR NEOPLASIA

Both adenocarcinoma *in situ* and invasive adenocarcinoma of the cervix are recognised but the relationship between these two conditions is much less clearly defined than is that between CIN and squamous carcinoma of the cervix. Adenocarcinomas currently constitute between 12% and 16% of all cervical neoplasms and this proportion is rising. Whether this reflects a genuine increase in the incidence of these tumours or is due to a reduction in the number of squamous carcinomas is uncertain.

Many adenocarcinomas are found in women with aetiological factors similar to those for squamous carcinoma, and HPV strains 16 and 18 have been identified in adenocarcinomas.

ADENOCARCINOMA *IN SITU*

Adenocarcinoma *in situ* occurs in the mucus-secreting columnar epithelium on the surface of a cervical ectopy, within the endocervical canal or within endocervical crypts. It is recognised histologically by:

- Stratification of the epithelial cells.
- Loss of nuclear polarity, loss of mucin-secreting capacity.
- An increase in nucleo-cytoplasmic ratios, cellular pleomorphism, nuclear hyperchromatism.
- The presence of numerous, sometimes atypical, mitoses (Figure 3.10).

An increasing complexity of the glandular pattern is often, although not invariably, present. The least well-differentiated forms come to resemble squamous CIN 3. Lesser degrees of epithelial abnormality are recognised, to which the term 'cervical glandular intraepithelial neoplasia' (CGIN or GIN) is sometimes applied. This is intended to make the terminology comparable to that of the squamous lesions but it is not yet in common usage.

The relationship between adenocarcinoma *in situ* and invasive adenocarcinoma of the cervix and the risk of progression from one to the other is not established. In certain cases, the origin of an adenocarcinoma from an *in situ* lesion can be traced but an accompanying adenocarcinoma *in situ* is not necessarily identified adjacent to all adenocarcinomas. The clinical significance of CGIN is currently unknown.

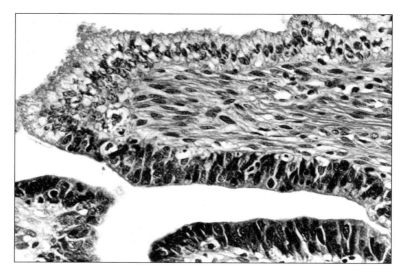

Figure 3.10 Adenocarcinoma *in situ* of the cervix. The crypt at the top of the field is lined by normal mucus-secreting columnar endocervical epithelium. In contrast, the lower crypt is lined with cells showing high nucleo-cytoplasmic ratios, large hyperchromatic nuclei and diminished mucin secretion.

ADENOCARCINOMA

There are several histological types of adenocarcinoma, of which by far the most common is the endocervical type in which the constituent cells bear an anarchic resemblance to those of the normal endocervix.

Endocervical adenocarcinoma

These tumours may be well, moderately well, or poorly differentiated. The well-differentiated tumours form glandular acini and branching clefts and crypts and the cells resemble those of the endocervix to a greater or lesser extent (Figure 3.11). Loss of differentiation is characterised by the loss of the glandular pattern and mucus-secreting capacity. The least well-differentiated forms assume a solid rather than a glandular pattern and thus come, histologically, to resemble a squamous carcinoma with which they may be confused.

Some endocervical adenocarcinomas are extremely well differentiated and have a surprisingly bland histological appearance. They are known as 'minimal deviation adenocarcinomas' or as 'adenoma malignum'.

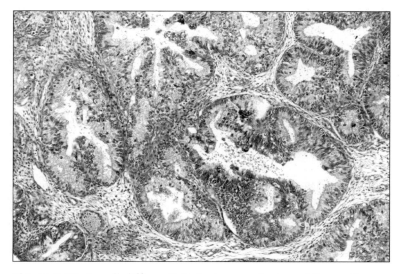

Figure 3.11 A well-differentiated adenocarcinoma of the cervix. The tumour is composed of well-formed glandular acini lined by tall mucus-secreting columnar epithelium which is similar to that of the normal endocervix.

Clear-cell carcinoma

Cervical neoplasms of this type are identical to the clear-cell adenocarcinoma of the vagina and, although occurring typically in DES-exposed girls, are by no means limited to this group.

Endometrioid adenocarcinoma

This term is used to describe carcinomas which are identical histologically with those adenocarcinomas that develop in the endometrium. They are uncommon in the cervix.

Rare cervical adenocarcinomas

These include the papillary serous adenocarcinoma, which is histologically identical to a papillary serous adenocarcinoma of the ovary; enteric adenocarcinomas, which resemble intestinal adenocarcinomas and are probably derived from foci of gastrointestinal metaplasia and mesonephric adenocarcinomas which arise from remnants of the mesonephric duct.

CARCINOMA OF MIXED PATTERN

About eight to ten percent of cervical carcinomas show evidence of

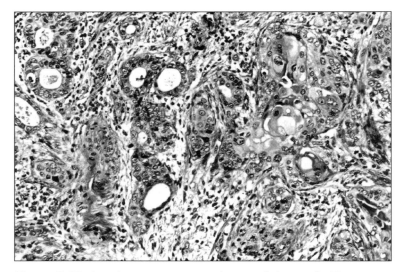

Figure 3.12 An adenosquamous carcinoma of the cervix. The tumour has two distinct, though intermingled, components. To the left there are well-formed infiltrating glandular acini, whilst to the right there is a focally-keratinising squamous cell carcinoma.

differentiation along more than one cell line. Most commonly these are adenosquamous carcinomas (Figure 3.12) and the diagnosis is made only when histological examination of the tumour is carried out, as they are similar in gross appearance to squamous and adenocarcinomas. These are aggressive neoplasms with a rather poor prognosis.

SMALL-CELL CARCINOMAS

These neoplasms constitute about two percent of cases of malignant cervical disease and occur most commonly in the fifth decade of life. They are of neuroendocrine origin and are highly aggressive tumours.

4 The endometrium

Histology of the endometrium

DURING THE MENSTRUAL CYCLE

During the follicular phase of the menstrual cycle (Figure 4.1) when oestrogen levels are rising, the various elements of the functional layer of the endometrium proliferate. The glands are at first straight and narrow but become slightly tortuous during the latter part of this phase, when the rate of glandular growth outstrips that of the stroma. The glands are lined by columnar cells with basally-situated nuclei and there may be a minor degree of multilayering in the late proliferative phase. The stroma is cellular and, because the stromal cells have little cytoplasm, often presents a 'naked-nuclei' appearance. Mitotic figures are present in both glands and stroma throughout the proliferative phase.

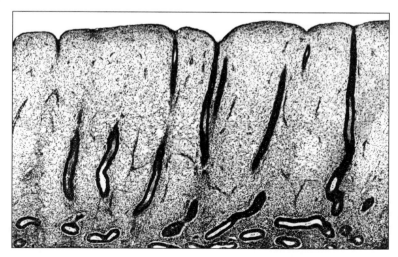

Figure 4.1 Endometrium in the early proliferative phase. The glands, which are straight and narrow, are set in a delicate cellular stroma.

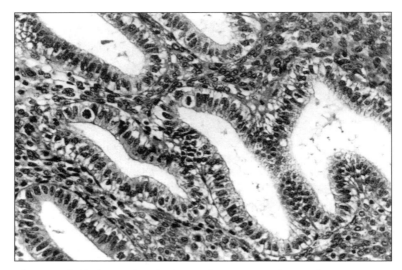

Figure 4.2 Endometrium in the early secretory phase. There are clear sub-nuclear vacuoles in the glandular epithelial cells.

In the average cycle, ovulation occurs at about the 14th day with the endometrium then entering, under the influence of the rising progesterone levels, the early secretory phase. The morphological changes that characterise the early secretory phase take 24–36 hours to develop. The glands increase slightly in diameter during this period and become somewhat more tortuous. Mitotic figures are still present in the glandular epithelium but decrease progressively in number as progesterone exerts its anti-oestrogen effect. The defining feature of the early secretory phase, clearly apparent 48 hours after ovulation, is the appearance of glycogen-containing subnuclear vacuoles in the glands (Figure 4.2). These vacuoles, when numerous and prominent, are taken as being definite evidence that ovulation has occurred. The early secretory phase lasts for about four days and between the fifth and ninth post-ovulatory days the endometrium is in the mid-secretory phase of the cycle (Figure 4.3). The subnuclear vacuoles move to a supranuclear position and secrete their contents into the gland lumina, the nuclei of the glands returning to a basal position. Glandular secretion is at a peak during this period and the glands become increasingly dilated and tortuous.

During the mid-secretory phase the stroma is markedly oedematous, largely because of the hormonally-induced increases in both bloodflow through, and hydrostatic pressure in, the endometrial capillary complexes.

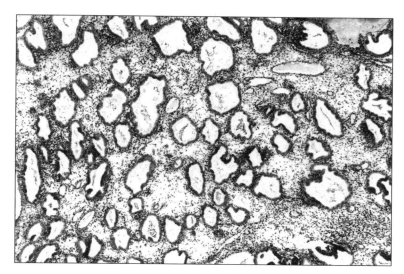

Figure 4.3 Endometrium in the mid-secretory phase. The glands are distended by secretions and are rather angular: the stroma is oedematous.

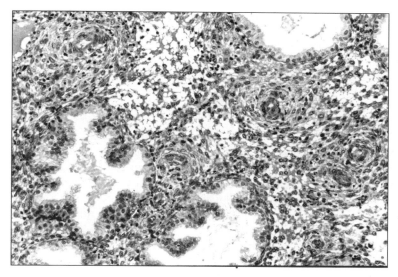

Figure 4.4 Endometrium in the late secretory phase. The glands have a serrated outline, having collapsed after secreting their contents, and the spiral arteries, which are cuffed by decidualised stromal cells, are prominent.

At the 11th post-ovulatory day the endometrium passes into the late secretory phase (Figure 4.4). Glandular secretion diminishes and the glands tend to collapse and become increasingly tortuous. The stromal oedema regresses and the stromal cells take on a pre-decidual appearance, becoming plump with abundant acidophilic cytoplasm and small nuclei. The pre-decidual cells appear first as a mantle around the spiral arteries which, after being previously inconspicuous, are now well developed and prominent. Later, pre-decidual change is seen in the cells surrounding the glands and in those lying directly below the surface epithelium. Towards the end of the late secretory phase the stroma consists largely of sheets of pre-decidual cells which are infiltrated by neutrophil polymorphonuclear leucocytes and by granulated lymphocytes (K cells). The leucocytes increase in number as the endometrium undergoes menstrual changes, characterised by crumbling, necrosis, glandular collapse and haemorrhage.

It will be appreciated that throughout the proliferative phase of the cycle the endometrium shows a rather inconsistent pattern and thus an accurate estimation of the day of the menstrual cycle is not possible. After ovulation the endometrium shows an orderly pattern of time-related changes which allows for a relatively precise estimate, to within 24–48 hours, of the stage of the cycle.

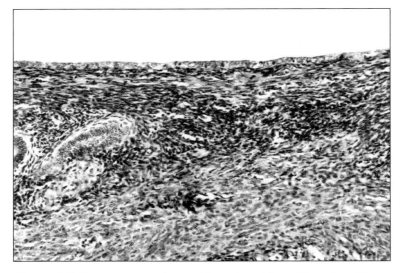

Figure 4.5 Postmenopausal atrophic endometrium. There is neither secretory nor proliferative activity. The glands are narrow and the stroma is compact.

AFTER THE MENOPAUSE

Oestrogen levels diminish quite abruptly in many women at the time of the menopause and this results in endometrial atrophy, the endometrium becoming shallow, the glands small and inactive and the stroma compact (Figure 4.5). In some women, however, oestrogen levels show a more gradual decline and there may be a rather irregular pattern of proliferation, with mitotic activity still being discernible for up to two years after cessation of ovulation. Gradually, however, this low-grade stimulation ceases and the presence of mitotic figures in the endometrium more than three years after the menopause is a clear indication of either an abnormal source of endogenous oestrogens or the administration of exogenous oestrogens.

In a high proportion of postmenopausal women the endometrial glands are, either focally or diffusely, cystically dilated (Figure 4.6), such glands being lined by a single layer of flattened epithelial cells. The incidence of such cystic change increases progressively with advancing age and it is clear that this is because of blockage of gland ducts during the process of endometrial atrophy and condensation. The cystically-dilated glands may, on occasion, become polypoid.

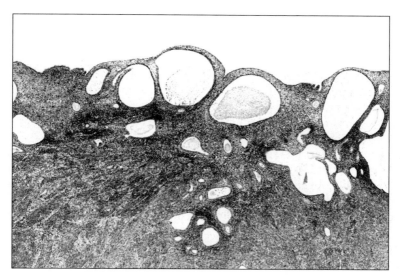

Figure 4.6 Senile cystic change in an atrophic postmenopausal endometrium. Some of the glands are cystically dilated and are lined by an attenuated epithelium: there is neither proliferative nor secretory activity.

Functional abnormalities of the endometrium

It is usual to distinguish between those abnormalities of endometrial morphology which are secondary to hormonal disturbances and are sometimes known as functional disorders of the endometrium, although the term has little to commend it, and those in which there is a primary disease process within the endometrium.

Functional abnormalities of the endometrium fall into two main groups, those in which there are inadequacies of hormonal stimulation and those in which such stimulation is excessive.

LOW OESTROGEN STATES

In the absence of ovarian follicular development there is no oestrogen secretion and hence an absence of endometrial growth and proliferation. In such women, the endometrium is shallow and inactive and the uterus is lined only by endometrium of basal type. This is normal after the menopause but is seen in such pathological processes as gonadal dysgenesis, premature menopause, 17-hydroxylase deficiency, gonadotrophin-resistant ovary syndrome and hypogonadotrophic hypogonadism.

HIGH OESTROGEN STATES

The secretory phase of the menstrual cycle is remarkably constant at 14 days and most variation in cycle length is due to changes in the length of the proliferative or follicular phase which is considered to be abnormally long only when it exceeds 21 days. The endometrium in such cycles may be of normal appearance or show nothing more than an increased stratification of the glandular epithelium and a mild increase in volume of the endometrium; there are no significant consequences of these minor changes. There will, however, be less frequent menstruation than normal and the periods may be irregular.

In some circumstances ovarian follicular development is not followed by ovulation. As a consequence of continued oestrogen secretion by the developing follicle or follicles, the endometrium will continue to grow in an uninterrupted fashion and will eventually become hyperplastic. This condition is discussed in more detail below.

LOW PROGESTERONE STATES

Low progesterone states are a natural consequence of failure of normal follicular maturation and of ovulation. In some women, however, less profound deficiencies occur as normal ovulation is followed by inadequate development of the corpus luteum with resulting progesterone deficiency. These patients, described as having 'luteal phase insufficiency' or 'inadequate secretory phase', complain of a variety of symptoms, amongst which the most common are premenstrual spotting (the loss of small amounts of blood), prolonged menstruation and infertility.

Progesterone deficiency may affect the endometrium in one of the following ways:

1 A delay in the development of secretory changes following ovulation, so that the endometrium appears to be less mature than suggested by the date of the woman's cycle.
2 A discrepancy between the maturation of the glands and stroma, with the stroma appearing to be more mature than the glands.
3 A variable degree of secretory change in different glands in the same tissue, also known as 'irregular ripening' (Figure 4.7).

EXOGENOUS HORMONE EFFECTS

Many of the functional abnormalities of the endometrium may be mimicked by exogenous hormones given to a patient for therapeutic or contraceptive purposes. Thus the administration of oestrogen, unopposed by a progestogen, may result in the development of a simple, complex, or atypical endometrial hyperplasia or even a carcinoma.

Progestogens may so inhibit endogenous oestrogenic activity that

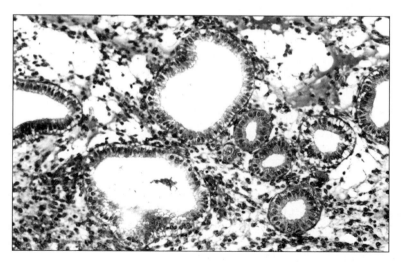

Figure 4.7 Luteal phase insufficiency: irregular ripening. The glands in this field vary in their degree of maturation. Those to the left are large and show appearances consistent with the fourth to fifth postovulatory day. The glands to the right are small, some showing no evidence of secretory change and others showing early secretory change.

the endometrium can eventually become shallow and atrophic.

The changes in the endometrium which accompany the use of a combined steroid contraceptive pill vary greatly according to the dose of hormone administered, the relative potency of the steroids included in the combination or their duration of use. The appearances may mimic those of luteal phase insufficiency or resemble those seen after administration of a progestogen.

Inflammation and infection in the endometrium

The endometrium normally contains a population of lymphocytes and, at the time of menstruation, polymorphonuclear leucocytes. The presence of such cells in the endometrium is therefore not indicative of an inflammatory process. Plasma cells, eosinophils, tissue breakdown associated with a polymorphonuclear leucocyte infiltrate at times other than at menstruation, granulomas and lymphoid aggregates with germinal centres are, however, not normally found in the endometrium and are regarded as hallmarks of inflammation.

NON-INFECTIVE INFLAMMATION

Inflammation which is not infective in origin may be physiological, such as that which accompanies the remodelling of the decidua in the early stages of pregnancy or following delivery or it may be pathological. The latter type occurs when there is abnormal tissue breakdown in the uterine cavity, for example when there is torsion of a polyp, in association with an IUCD, when there is prolonged and frequent heavy bleeding or in the presence of neoplasms.

INFECTION OF THE ENDOMETRIUM

Endometrial infections are uncommon because the establishment of an infective lesion is discouraged by the efficient downwards drainage of the uterine cavity, the regular shedding of the endometrium which occurs in the reproductive years and by the presence of an effective cervical mucus barrier which prevents the ascent of most organisms into the uterus from the cervix and vagina.

If, however, these natural protective mechanisms are disturbed, endometritis may supervene. Thus, drainage from the uterine cavity may be partly or completely obstructed by polyps, neoplasms, or retained products of conception within the uterine cavity, by acute flexion of the uterus, by scarring of the cervix following surgery, obstetric trauma, or radiotherapy, or by a cervical neoplasm. Disruption of the cervical mucus barrier occurs in patients with chronic cervical infection, in whom mucus secretion may be impaired; in women in whom previous cervical surgery has removed much of the mucus-secreting tissue; and in women who have had operative procedures involving dilatation or biopsy of the cervix. The mucus barrier does not offer complete protection, as certain organisms such as *Neisseria gonorrhoeae* are capable of penetrating it. Interruption of endometrial shedding, for reasons other than pregnancy, does not in itself predispose to infection but permits any infection that may occur to become established.

The uterus has little natural protection against those infections which spread via the bloodstream or descend from the fallopian tubes.

Pathological features of endometrial inflammation

Inflammation may be acute, subacute, or chronic and chronic inflammatory lesions may be granulomatous or non-granulomatous. Acute endometritis is recognised by the presence, in the endometrium, of polymorphonuclear leucocytes associated with tissue destruction at times other than at menstruation. Acute infections are usually polymicrobial and occur most commonly following abortion, although an acute endometritis may be due to gonococcal infection.

In an active chronic endometrial inflammation (Figure 4.8) plasma cells, polymorphonuclear leucocytes, lymphocytes and histiocytes are found in the stroma and polymorphonuclear leucocytes are present in the glandular lumens. If inflammation is particularly severe, there may be disturbances in the induction of hormone receptors, as a consequence of which the tissue may fail to reflect the normal cyclical hormonal changes.

The incidence of chronic non-granulomatous endometritis is difficult to determine and almost certainly underestimated because of the difficulty in distinguishing an abnormal diffuse chronic inflammatory cell infiltrate from the normal lymphocytic population of the endometrium. When the inflammatory infiltrate is predominantly histiocytic the term histiocytic or xanthomatous endometritis is sometimes used.

Chronic granulomatous inflammation in the endometrium is regarded as being due to tuberculosis until otherwise proven and, indeed, non-tuberculous granulomatous inflammation is extremely uncommon. Endometrial tuberculosis is almost always secondary to infection in the fallopian tubes, from which site there is repeated inoculation of the endometrial surface. The regular menstrual shedding of the endometrium tends to prevent establishment of infection and, because the shedding of the endometrium occurs at about the same interval as the time taken for a granuloma to be recognisable histologically, granulomas tend to be small and poorly developed (Figure 4.9).

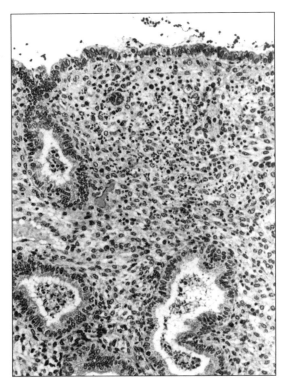

Figure 4.8 Active chronic inflammation of the endometrium. The endometrial stroma is infiltrated by neutrophils, lymphocytes and plasma cells and the glands contain an acute inflammatory cell exudate.

Figure 4.9 Endometrial tuberculosis. There are non-caseating granulomas with epithelioid macrophages and Langerhans' giant cells centrally, whilst peripherally there is a cuff of lymphocytes.

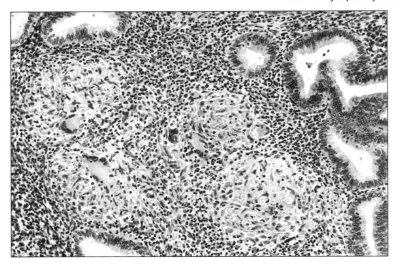

Caseation is rarely seen unless endometrial shedding has been incomplete, when caseating granulomas may be seen in the basal endometrium, or after the menopause when extensive, confluent, caseating endometrial tuberculosis may be encountered.

Consequences of endometrial inflammation

Acute inflammation has no long-term adverse effects unless infection persists, there is secondary infection, or infection spreads to the fallopian tubes.

When inflammation is so severe that there is structural damage to the basal layers of the endometrium, tissue regrowth may be hampered, a condition known as Asherman's syndrome. When this happens the stroma may be extensively replaced by fibrous tissue, intrauterine adhesions may be formed and the glands may be unresponsive to normal hormonal stimulation.

Endometrial metaplasia

The tissue of the Müllerian system, that is, the fallopian tubes, uterus and endocervix, retain into adulthood a capacity to differentiate into one or more of the tissues to which the paracoelomic epithelium, the embryonic precursor of the Müllerian tract, gives rise during fetal development. In the adult, this takes the form of epithelial metaplasia which, in the endometrium, is characterised by replacement of the epithelial lining of one or more glands, completely or partly, by a squamous, serous, or mucinous epithelium (Figure 4.10). This is most common in hyperoestrogenic states and in the elderly, postmenopausal woman. In older patients with cervical obstruction and intrauterine infection, the uterus may become lined only by squamous epithelium, a condition known as 'ichthyosis uteri' and one which may occasionally give rise to a squamous cell carcinoma. Focal intraglandular squamous metaplasia also occurs in adenocarcinomas of the endometrium and is discussed below. Endometrial stromal metaplasia, with bone, cartilage or smooth muscle formation, also occurs but is extremely uncommon.

Endometrial polyps

The term 'endometrial polyp' could be used to describe any polypoidal lesion protruding into the uterine cavity. By convention, however, the term is restricted to non-neoplastic pedunculated or sessile nodules composed of either functional or basal endometrium or a combination of the two.

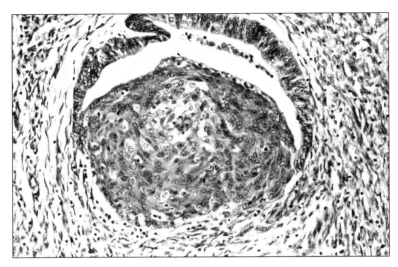

Figure 4.10 Intraglandular squamous metaplasia of the endometrium. A focus of bland metaplastic squamous epithelium replaces part of the lining of this endometrial gland and protrudes into the lumen.

Endometrial polyps develop as a consequence of focal stromal and glandular overgrowth. It is believed that a focal hypersensitivity to oestrogen or lack of sensitivity to progesterone may allow a portion of endometrium to remain unshed at the end of menstruation. This focus continues to grow in each successive cycle until it protrudes into the uterine cavity. Polyps do not occur before the menarche, are most common in the fifth decade of life and are sometimes encountered in postmenopausal women.

Endometrial polyps vary greatly, ranging from small lesions discovered incidentally to large masses which protrude from the cervical os. They may be sessile or pedunculated. In the reproductive years they are usually composed either of non-functional basal endometrium or have a central core of basal-type endometrium containing thick-walled arteries covered by a layer of functional endometrium of variable thickness (Figure 4.11). The latter is frequently out of step with the endometrium elsewhere in the uterine cavity, for example showing only weak proliferative activity during the follicular phase and either lacking secretory features or showing only weak or patchy secretory activity in the luteal phase. The tip of the polyp is often congested, even to the naked eye, and focally inflamed. Ulceration may occur and the surface epithelium may undergo squamous metaplasia, this being

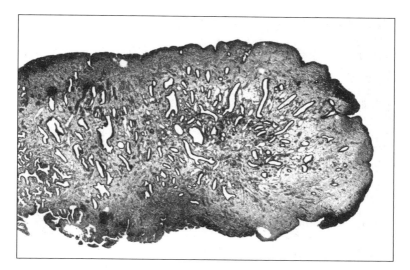

Figure 4.11 An endometrial polyp. This is composed of gland-containing endometrial tissue.

seen particularly in those polyps protruding from the cervical os or developing from the uterine isthmus. On rare occasions pedunculated polyps may undergo torsion and infarction. Polyps in postmenopausal women may be formed either of inactive basal-type endometrium or of senile cystic endometrium with a fibrous stroma.

Polyps commonly recur, presumably because they have been incompletely removed or because the underlying defect persists. Polyps do not predispose to the development of a carcinoma. Malignant change occasionally occurs in polyps but most apparent instances of this phenomenon have actually been adenocarcinomas growing in a polypoidal fashion.

Endometrial hyperplasia

Endometrial hyperplasia is widely regarded as a possible precursor of endometrial adenocarcinoma. The term 'endometrial hyperplasia' encompasses, however, several distinct conditions and it is important to distinguish between those types of hyperplasia associated with a significant risk of evolving into an adenocarcinoma and those devoid of any such risk. The defining feature of an endometrial hyperplasia which is indicative of a propensity for malignant change is cytological atypia. Any hyperplastic lesion of the endometrium showing this abnormality is classed as 'atypical hyperplasia'. Hyperplastic conditions that lack cytological atypia are divided into 'simple' and 'complex' forms.

SIMPLE ENDOMETRIAL HYPERPLASIA

Simple hyperplasia (also often, but incorrectly, called cystic glandular hyperplasia) is a relatively common condition and represents the physiological response of the endometrium to prolonged, unopposed oestrogenic stimulation, being in fact only one component of a generalised hyperplasia of all the uterine tissues. The endometrium is thickened and often polypoidal. The entire endometrium is involved and, histologically, there is a loss of the normal distinction between basal and functional zones. The endometrial glands show a proliferative pattern but vary markedly in calibre, some being unusually wide, others of normal calibre and yet others unduly narrow (Figure 4.12). The glandular epithelium is formed by plump cuboidal or low columnar cells with basophilic cytoplasm and round, centrally- or basally-situated nuclei. The endometrial stroma shares in the hyperplastic process and hence the gland-to-stroma ratio is normal with no glandular crowding. The stroma appears hypercellular whilst mitotic figures, present in both glands and stroma, may be sparse or abundant but are invariably of normal form.

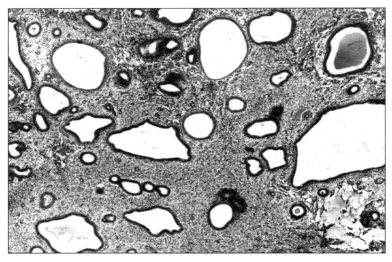

Figure 4.12 Simple endometrial hyperplasia. The endometrium contains glands of various calibre, some being unduly small, others of normal size and yet others which are dilated.

Simple hyperplasia may complicate exogenous oestrogen therapy, oestrogenic ovarian tumours, or the polycystic ovary syndrome. The commonest cause of the condition is, however, a series of anovulatory cycles in which oestrogen production by persistent ovarian follicles is not opposed by any luteal secretion of progesterone. Hence this type of hyperplasia occurs most commonly in the perimenarchal and perimenopausal years, when anovulatory cycles are common. If ovulatory cycles are resumed or if a progestogen is administered, a simple hyperplasia will regress and the endometrium will rapidly return to its normal state.

Simple endometrial hyperplasia is, in our opinion, not a precursor of, and does not evolve into, atypical endometrial hyperplasia and is not associated with any increased risk of developing an adenocarcinoma.

COMPLEX HYPERPLASIA

This may occur under the same circumstances as does simple hyperplasia, that is in an endometrium exposed to unopposed oestrogenic stimulation, but it can also develop in a normally cycling or atrophic endometrium. A complex hyperplasia is restricted to the glandular component of the endometrium and does not involve the stroma. It is usually focal or multifocal in nature, involving only a group, or groups, of glands. The hyperplastic glands are variable in size, often larger than normal and are crowded together with a reduction in the amount of intervening stroma. The involved glands show an abnormal pattern of growth with outpouchings or buddings of the glandular epithelium in the stroma to give a 'finger-in-glove' pattern (Figure 4.13). Intraluminal epithelial tufting is also common. The glandular epithelium is regular and formed of cuboidal or columnar cells with basal or central nuclei and there is no cytological atypia.

The risk of a complex hyperplasia evolving into an adenocarcinoma has not been fully determined but is almost certainly extremely low.

ATYPICAL HYPERPLASIA

This lesion develops under the same circumstances as does a complex hyperplasia, some cases being 'oestrogen driven' and others occurring in the absence of undue oestrogenic stimulation of the endometrium. As with a complex hyperplasia, only the glands are hyperplastic and the lesions are either focal or multifocal.

In the hyperplastic areas (Figure 4.14) there is crowding of the glands with a marked reduction in intervening stroma. In severe cases the glands show a 'back-to-back' pattern, the stroma between the glands being reduced to a thin wisp or completely obliterated. The

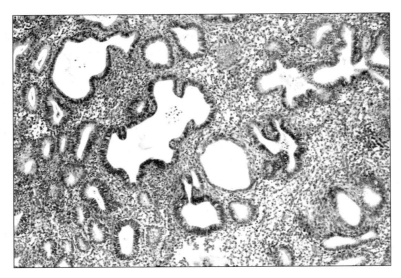

Figure 4.13 Complex hyperplasia of the endometrium. The endometrial glands are more closely packed than normal and are irregular in outline.

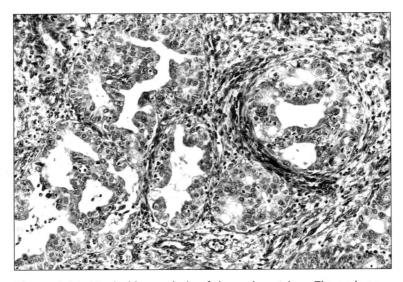

Figure 4.14 Atypical hyperplasia of the endometrium. The endometrial glands are closely packed, irregular in outline and lined by cells showing enlarged nuclei: the lining epithelium shows loss of polarity and stratification.

glands are usually irregular in shape and are lined by cells showing varying degrees of atypia. In the milder forms of atypical hyperplasia the epithelial nuclei tend to be ovoid with retention of polarity and of a near normal chromatin pattern, however much the nucleo-cytoplasmic ratio has increased. In more severe cases the nuclei are round and enlarged, nuclear polarity is lost, nucleoli are increased in size and there is an abnormal chromatin pattern. With progressing severity of atypia there is an increasing degree of epithelial multi-layering and of intraluminal tufting.

An atypical hyperplasia can undoubtedly evolve into an endometrial adenocarcinoma. The exact magnitude of this risk is not adequately defined, but a reasonable estimate would be that approximately 25% of cases of atypical endometrial hyperplasia will eventually give rise to an invasive endometrial adenocarcinoma. When considering this progression from an atypical hyperplasia to an invasive neoplasm it is widely assumed that the controlled proliferation of a hyperplastic process may 'slip over' into the cellular anarchy of neoplasia. It must be doubted, however, if this is a viable concept and there are good grounds for believing that the lesion classed as an atypical hyperplasia of the endometrium is a form of intraendometrial neoplasia, compa-rable in many respects to CIN. The fact that many cases of atypical hyperplasia will regress if treated with a progestogen does not conflict with this hypothesis.

Malignant epithelial tumours of the endometrium

ADENOCARCINOMA

The vast majority of endometrial neoplasms are adenocarcinomas, which develop most commonly during the sixth decade, many patients being in the early postmenopausal years. Only about five percent of these neoplasms occur in premenopausal women.

It is traditionally maintained that women who develop endometrial adenocarcinoma are commonly nulliparous, often have an unusually late menopause and have a high incidence of hypertension, diabetes mellitus and obesity. The association of this neoplasm with nulliparity and a late menopause has withstood the test of case-control studies but there is considerable doubt as to whether there is any real link with either hypertension or diabetes. It is certain, however, that obese women have a significantly increased risk of developing an endome-trial adenocarcinoma.

The role of oestrogens in the pathogenesis of endometrial adenocar-cinoma has been much debated but it is now well established that the administration of exogenous oestrogens is associated with a greatly increased risk of developing endometrial adenocarcinoma. In the USA, the rise of incidence of this neoplasm which occurred after the introduction of widespread unopposed oestrogen hormonal replacement therapy occurred rapidly. This suggests that under these circumstances oestrogens were acting as a promoter substance, exposure to a presumed initiator mechanism being therefore very common.

It is thus established that oestrogens can be implicated in the pathogenesis of some endometrial adenocarcinoma. It remains uncertain however, whether an overproduction of endogenous oestrogen is of aetiological importance in those women who form the vast majority of cases and who develop endometrial adenocarcinoma in the absence of exogenous hormones. It is certainly true that patients with oestrogen-secreting ovarian tumours have a notably high incidence of associated endometrial adenocarcinoma, but such cases represent only a tiny minority. Many women with endometrial adenocarcinoma have, however, an increased ability to convert androstenedione, of adrenal origin, into oestrone. This conversion occurs principally in the fat cells of the body and this is probably why obese women, with their excess number of fat cells, are particularly subject to endometrial neoplasia. A similar oestrone excess would, of course, result as a consequence of a primary overproduction of androstenedione and it is therefore of particular note that women with untreated polycystic ovary syndrome (PCOS), in which there is excessive ovarian synthesis of androstenedione, suffer not only a high incidence of adenocarcinoma but tend to develop the neoplasm at an unusually early age.

Even taking into account the above factors, it is clear that by no means all endometrial adenocarcinomas are oestrogen-related. A significant proportion of these neoplasms arise in an atrophic endometrium and these are probably not oestrogen-driven. The pathogenesis of such tumours is obscure, but it is of note that they often appear to be more aggressive than are those which occur in a setting of hyperoestrogenism.

An endometrial adenocarcinoma may appear as a localised plaque, polyp, or nodule, usually in the upper part of the uterus. More commonly the tumour presents as a diffuse nodular or polypoidal thickening of the uterine lining or as a bulky friable mass which fills, or even distends, the uterine cavity.

Histologically, most endometrial adenocarcinomas show a greater or lesser degree of endometrial differentiation and are classed as 'endometrioid adenocarcinomas'. Many are well differentiated and bear a resemblance, albeit an anarchic one, to normal proliferative endometrium (Figure 4.15). They are formed of irregular, tightly-packed, convoluted glandular acini lined by columnar cells showing a

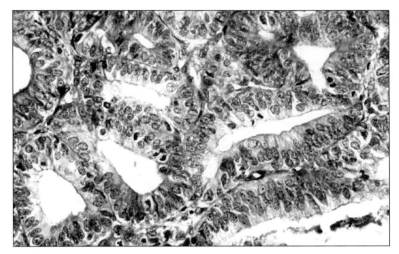

Figure 4.15 A well-differentiated adenocarcinoma of the endometrium. The neoplasm is composed of closely-packed, well-formed glandular acini lined by highly abnormal cells in which mitoses are frequent.

variable degree of pleomorphism, nuclear hyperchromatism and mitotic activity, commonly with irregular multilayering and intraluminal tufting. The stroma is scanty and in many cases obliterated. Foci of necrosis, haemorrhage and leucocytic infiltration are common and there may be a noteworthy accumulation of foamy stromal histiocytes. Less well-differentiated endometrioid adenocarcinomas grow in a more solid fashion and grading of these neoplasms is based upon a consideration of both the proportion of the tumour showing a solid growth pattern and the degree of cytological atypia.

A number of histological variants of endometrial adenocarcinoma merit attention. Most endometrioid adenocarcinomas contain foci of bland squamous metaplasia and it has been suggested that those tumours in which such metaplasia is a prominent feature should be put into a separate category of 'adenoacanthoma'. The frequency with which squamous metaplasia occurs, the subjectivity in deciding what is meant by 'prominent' and the fact that squamous metaplasia, even if widespread, does not alter the prognosis for any given adenocarcinoma, have led to the abandonment of the adenoacanthomas as a diagnostic category.

Papillary serous carcinomas, a form of endometrial adenocarcinoma (Figure 4.16), resemble a tubal adenocarcinoma. Neoplasms of this type may arise in foci of endometrial tubal metaplasia or from uncom-

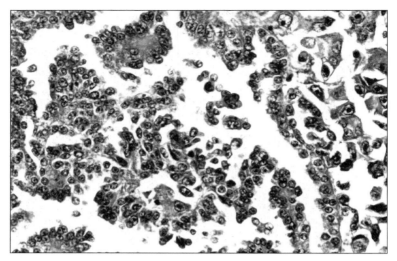

Figure 4.16 A serous papillary adenocarcinoma of the endometrium. The tumour is composed of papillary and more solid areas formed by cells which are poorly differentiated but of tubal type.

mitted Müllerian cells which pursue a tubal, rather than an endometrial, pathway of differentiation. The latter cells can also differentiate along endocervical lines and thus give rise to the rare mucinous adenocarcinomas of the endometrium.

Clear-cell adenocarcinomas, identical histologically to clear-cell neoplasms of the vagina and ovary (Figure 4.17), also occur in the endometrium.

Well-differentiated endometrioid adenocarcinomas tend to be slowly growing and often remain within the confines of the uterus for a considerable time, spreading initially by direct invasion of the myometrium and cervix. Later the neoplasm may penetrate the uterine serosa and seed into the pouch of Douglas and on to the pelvic peritoneum. Cornual carcinomas commonly extend into the fallopian tubes and tumour cells may pass through the tubal ostia to be deposited on the ovaries and pelvic peritoneum. Local spread may also involve the broad ligament and the parametrium. Lymphatic spread occurs to pelvic and para-aortic nodes, whilst haematogenous dissemination to lungs, liver, adrenals and bones occurs late. It should be stressed that this slow pattern of growth is only a feature of the well-differentiated endometrioid tumours. Serous papillary and clear-cell carcinomas pursue a much more aggressive course with early deep penetration of the myometrium and spread to para-aortic nodes.

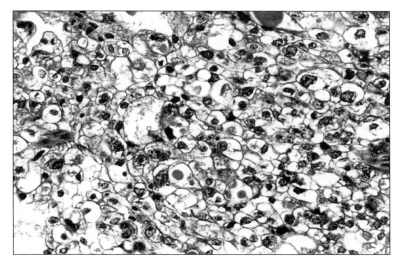

Figure 4.17 Clear-cell adenocarcinoma. The tumour is composed of cells with well-demarcated margins, large nuclei and copious clear cytoplasm.

The overall five-year survival for women with endometrial adenocarcinoma is about 65%. Stage is clearly of prognostic importance but other features related to survival are the grade of the neoplasm and the histological type, papillary serous tumours and clear-cell adenocarcinomas having, as already remarked, a poor prognosis. Other prognostic factors to be taken into account are those indicative of a poor outlook, namely:

- Deep invasion of the myometrium.
- The presence of tumour cells in vascular spaces.
- A lack of oestrogen and progesterone receptors.
- An aneuploid DNA pattern.

A further point of some importance is that tumours arising from a background of atypical hyperplasia have a better prognosis than do those developing in an atrophic endometrium.

ADENOSQUAMOUS CARCINOMA

These tumours, which account for about five percent of endometrial neoplasms, contain an admixture of both adenocarcinoma and squamous cell carcinoma (Figure 4.18). They differ from an adenocarcinoma with squamous metaplasia in so far as the squamous tissue is clearly malignant and invasive. Adenosquamous carcinomas tend to

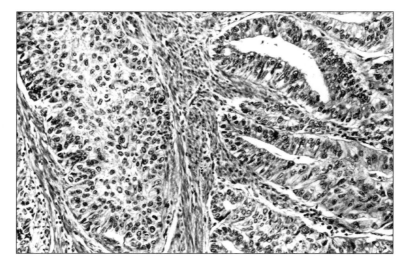

Figure 4.18 Adenosquamous carcinoma of the endometrium. Two distinct areas of tumour are seen. To the left, the tumour shows differentiation into squamous cell carcinoma whilst to the right there is adenocarcinomatous differentiation.

occur at a relatively late age and run an aggressive course, the five-year survival rate being below 40%.

SQUAMOUS CELL CARCINOMA

The endometrium is a rare site for this type of neoplasm which usually develops in elderly women with pyometra and complete squamous metaplasia of the surface epithelium (ichthyosis uteri). In younger patients CIN may spread upwards into the uterine body where it replaces the surface epithelium and can give rise to a squamous cell carcinoma. The prognosis for a squamous cell carcinoma of the endometrium is extremely poor.

Endometrial stromal sarcoma

Endometrial stromal sarcomas are formed of cells which resemble those of the endometrial stroma during the proliferative phase of the menstrual cycle. These neoplasms have traditionally been divided into low-grade and high-grade types, this distinction being based upon mitotic counts. It is now accepted, however, that most tumours classed as high-grade stromal sarcomas do not contain endometrial stromal-like cells and should be classed as undifferentiated uterine sarcomas. Furthermore, in cases that do meet the diagnostic criteria for an endometrial stromal neoplasm, mitotic counts are not of prognostic value and therefore the distinction between high-grade and low-grade endometrial stromal sarcomas is no longer valid.

Endometrial stromal sarcomas can form localised tumour masses but have a particular tendency to infiltrate the vascular and lymphatic channels of the myometrium extensively. Cords of tumour tissue may therefore protrude from the cut surface of the uterus, giving it a 'comedo' or 'rough towel' appearance. Histologically (Figure 4.19), the neoplasms are formed of sheets of spindle-shaped cells which resemble the endometrial stromal cells of the normal proliferative phase. Endometrial stromal sarcomas run an indolently malignant course, tend to spread into the parametrium and often recur locally, sometimes as long as 20 years after removal of the primary tumour. Approximately 20% of patients with these neoplasms will eventually succumb, usually after an extremely protracted course.

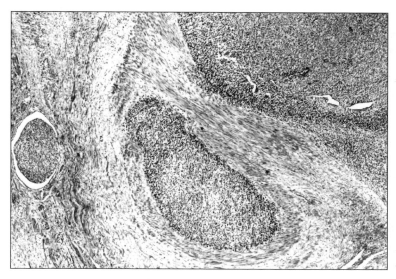

Figure 4.19 An endometrial stromal sarcoma of the uterus. The vascular spaces of the myometrium are permeated by a tumour composed of fairly regular uniform cells resembling those of the normal endometrial stroma.

Mixed tumours of the endometrium

Although most endometrial neoplasms are either purely epithelial or solely mesenchymal, a few show a dimorphic pattern and contain both epithelial and non-epithelial tissues. Such neoplasms, often classed as 'mixed Müllerian tumours', may be of low-grade malignancy and contain a benign epithelial component and a malignant mesenchymal element (adenosarcomas) or can be of high-grade malignancy with both epithelial and mesenchymal elements being malignant (carcinosarcoma). The epithelial component of a mixed tumour is usually of a type normally found in the Müllerian system but although the mesenchymal component commonly differentiates into either smooth muscle or endometrial stromal-like cells (that is, into tissues which are homologous for the uterus) it can also differentiate into tissue normally alien to the uterus, the most common of such heterologous elements being striated muscle, bone and cartilage.

Mixed tumours of high-grade malignancy, carcinosarcomas, are of unknown aetiology, occur principally in elderly women and form bulky, fleshy polypoid masses which fill the uterine cavity, sometimes extending into the endocervical canal and occasionally protruding through to the vagina. Histologically, they consist of an intimate admixture of carcinomatous and sarcomatous tissues (Figure 4.20). The adenocarcinomatous element usually resembles an endometrioid adenocarcinoma and the sarcomatous element is either undifferentiated or resembles an endometrial stromal sarcoma. Heterologous tissues may be present (Figure 4.21) but these are of no diagnostic or prognostic significance. Endometrial carcinosarcomas are highly aggressive neoplasms which tend to spread rapidly outside the uterus and metastasise via the bloodstream, the prognosis being generally poor.

The most important prognostic factor for these neoplasms, apart from stage, is the grade of the carcinomatous component. This fact, together with cytochemical and tissue culture findings, has led to the belief that carcinosarcomas are 'metaplastic carcinomas' or 'sarcomatoid carcinomas'.

Mixed tumours of low-grade malignancy, adenosarcomas, resemble macroscopically the carcinosarcomas but have a benign epithelial component, of endometrial, endocervical, or tubal type, set in a stroma resembling an endometrial stromal sarcoma. Heterologous elements may be present. The neoplasms spread outside the uterus in only about 50% of cases and distant metastases are very uncommon. Even women with spread outside the uterus (but limited to the pelvis) may survive for prolonged periods as this tumour pursues an indolently malignant course.

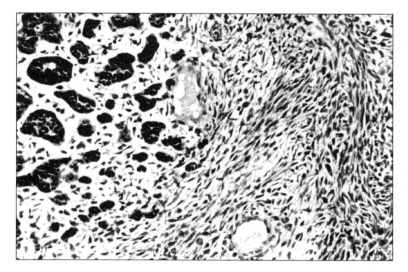

Figure 4.20 Carcinosarcoma of the endometrium. There is poorly-differentiated adenocarcinoma to the left and sarcoma to the right.

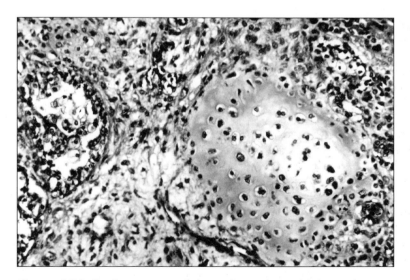

Figure 4.21 Carcinosarcoma of the endometrium with heterologous elements. An adenocarcinomatous gland is present to the left and the sarcomatous tissue, to the right, contains a focus of chondro-sarcoma.

5 The myometrium

Adenomyosis

This condition is characterised by the presence of endometrial tissue deep within the myometrium and there is almost invariably an associated hypertrophy of smooth muscle around the ectopic islands of endometrium. The foci of endometrial tissue may be distributed diffusely within the myometrium, in which case the uterus shows a roughly symmetrical enlargement, or can be focal, forming a poorly-defined tumour-like asymmetrical thickening of the myometrium. The localised form is often known as an 'adenomyoma', an unfortunate term because of its misleading connotation of neoplasia. Histologically, foci of adenomyosis consist of both endometrial glands and stroma (Figure 5.1). The glands are usually of basal type and thus do not show cyclic activity.

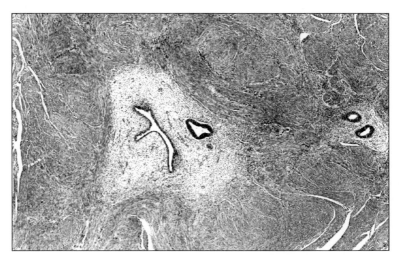

Figure 5.1 Adenomyosis. Within the myometrium there are two islands of endometrial tissue of basal type, both of which contain gland and stroma.

Adenomyosis is due to a down-growth of basal endometrium into the myometrium. Serial sectioning shows a continuity between the basal endometrium and foci of adenomyosis. The aetiology of this diverticular disease is, however, obscure, for although both curettage and oestrogenic stimulation have been proposed as aetiological factors, there is no proof that either is of causal significance.

Benign tumours

LEIOMYOMAS

These neoplasms are tumours of the smooth muscle cells of the myometrium. There is commonly an intermingling with fibrous tissue and the tumours are often inaccurately known as 'fibroids'. Myometrial leiomyomas are extremely common, being present in at least 25% of women above the age of 35 years and there is considerable circumstantial evidence that oestrogenic stimulation plays a role in their pathogenesis. Consequently, they develop only during the reproductive years, enlarge both during pregnancy and in women using contraceptive steroids and tend to shrink after the menopause.

The tumours are usually multiple and vary in size from tiny 'seedlings' to huge masses which fill the abdomen. They may be within the uterine wall (intramural), in a submucosal site immediately below the endometrium or may lie just below the peritoneal covering of the uterus in a subserosal site. Submucosal leiomyomas tend to bulge into and distort the uterine cavity, with thinning of the overlying endometrium. They sometimes become polypoid to form a mass which may fill the uterine cavity and can also extend through the endocervical canal into the vagina. Subserosal tumours may grow out from the uterine surface and can extend into the broad ligament. They may also become pedunculated, and such a neoplasm may, in rare cases, become attached to the omentum or pelvic peritoneum where, after losing its stalk, it derives a new blood supply and flourishes as a parasitic leiomyoma.

Uterine leiomyomas have a well-defined regular outline with a surrounding pseudocapsule of compressed muscle fibres. When sectioned they have a firm, bulging, white, whorled or trabeculated appearance. Histologically, they consist of smooth muscle fibres arranged in bundles and whorls (Figure 5.2). The cells are elongated with spindle- or cigar-shaped nuclei. Some tumours, known as cellular leiomyomas, contain densely-packed cells with elongated nuclei. Rarely, the smooth muscle cells are rounded with central nuclei and clear cytoplasm. Tumours containing such cells are classed as epithe-

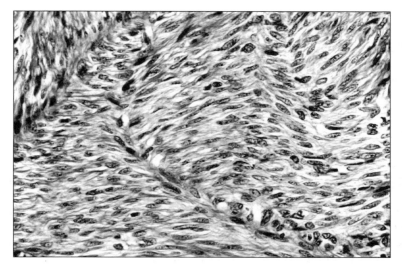

Figure 5.2 Uterine leiomyoma. The tumour is composed of interweaving bands of elongated smooth muscle cells. No mitotic figures are present.

lioid leiomyomas. Other variants of the usual pattern include the neurilemmoma-like leiomyoma, in which the nuclei show a pallisaded pattern; the symplastic leiomyoma, characterised by the presence of bizarre multinucleated cells and the leiomyoma with tubules in which an otherwise typical smooth muscle neoplasm contains epithelial-like tubules.

In all but the smallest leiomyomas degenerative changes tend to occur which are due to the neoplasm outgrowing its blood supply. Consequently, hyaline change, cystic change, myxoid degeneration, patchy necrosis and calcification are common. A pedunculated submucosal tumour may undergo torsion and infarction. A specific form of necrosis, seen particularly, but not only, in pregnancy, is 'red degeneration', characterised by a dull beefy-red appearance of the tumour which may also have a slightly fishy odour – this change can be accompanied by pain and fever and the presence of thrombosed vessels suggests that it represents haemorrhagic infarction of an extensively-hyalinised neoplasm.

Malignant change rarely occurs very rarely in uterine leiomyomas. However, certain variants of a leiomyoma, although histologically benign, do appear to behave in an invasive fashion. Thus, in the condition of 'intravenous leiomyomatosis' cords of smooth muscle are found in uterine and para-uterine veins, usually in association with more conventional leiomyomas elsewhere in the myometrium. The plugs of tumour cells occasionally extend as far as the inferior vena cava and can grow into the right atrium. It is not clear whether this condition is due to a special form of leiomyoma which, despite its benign nature, invades veins, or whether the tumours arise from the vein walls. A not dissimilar condition is benign metastasising leiomyoma, in which histologically benign uterine leiomyomas appear to be associated with pulmonary metastases which show no malignant features. Such cases probably represent the simultaneous independent development of pulmonary and uterine leiomyomas. In disseminated peritoneal leiomyomatosis, small leiomyomatous nodules are found scattered in the peritoneum and omentum in association with uterine leiomyomas. It is thought, however, that these extrauterine nodules arise *in situ* from the submesothelial mesenchyme of the peritoneum.

OTHER BENIGN TUMOURS

Fibromas, lipomas and haemangiomas can all occur in the myometrium but the only other benign myometrial neoplasm which is not of extreme rarity is the adenomatoid tumour. Neoplasms of this type are present in one percent of uteri and appear as small, rather poorly-delineated, masses in the cornual region, usually in an immediately subserosal site. Histologically (Figure 5.3), they are formed of

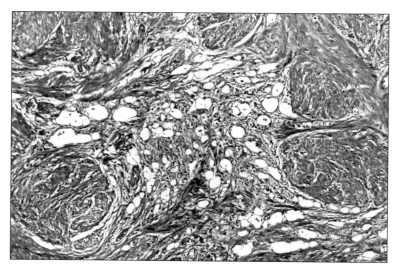

Figure 5.3 Adenomatoid tumour of the myometrium. The centre of the field is occupied by small gland-like spaces set in a fine fibrous stroma.

complex multiple gland-like spaces which are lined by a flattened or low cuboidal epithelium and are separated from each other by strands of fibromuscular tissue. Adenomatoid tumours are benign, almost invariably asymptomatic and are derived from the serosa, having all the characteristics of a benign mesothelioma.

Malignant neoplasms

LEIOMYOSARCOMA

These are rare, accounting for only one percent of malignant uterine neoplasms and occur most commonly in the fifth and sixth decades of life. The tumours are less well demarcated than are leiomyomas, often show areas of haemorrhage or necrosis and are characterised histologically by their cellularity, pleomorphism and high mitotic counts (Figure 5.4). Myometrial leiomyosarcomas spread locally to invade the pelvic organs but it is uncommon for lymph node metastases to occur. However, blood-borne spread to the lungs, liver and kidneys is common. The five-year survival rate for women with a neoplasm of this type is only 20–30%.

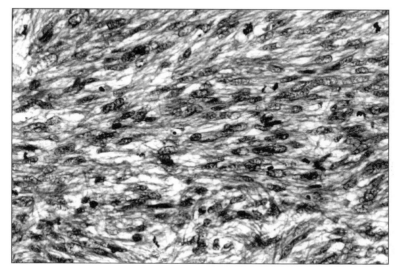

Figure 5.4 Leiomyosarcoma of the uterus. The neoplasm is composed of closely-packed smooth muscle cells with pleomorphic, hyperchromatic nuclei: there are many mitoses.

6 The fallopian tube

Inflammation of the fallopian tube

Inflammation of the fallopian tube (salpingitis), is a common disorder of the reproductive years. It is almost invariably infective, although minor degrees of irritative inflammation may occur as a response to the presence of necrotic tissue or blood in the tube due to, for example, menstrual reflux, bleeding from endometriotic foci, or the presence of an ectopic gestation. There may also be a mild inflammatory response to foreign bodies, such as those used in sterilisation procedures.

It is difficult to determine accurately the true incidence of infective salpingitis as most cases are not confirmed either histologically or bacteriologically at the time they present and depend only upon clinical criteria for their diagnosis, particularly in the acute phase.

The term 'pelvic inflammatory disease' (PID) is used to encompass signs and symptoms due to inflammation centred on the fallopian tube, but extending, in many cases, to involve the ovary, mesosalpinx, parametrium, uterine serosa and uterine ligaments. In the acute phase the clinical features are of an acute febrile illness associated with pelvic pain, vaginal discharge and tenderness over the fallopian tube. Chronic or subacute salpingitis may be recognised only when investigations for infertility are undertaken, this being a common complication of the disorder. It should be emphasised that the term PID refers only to a clinical concept and is one that should not be used as a pathological diagnosis.

Infection reaches the tube by one of three routes. Most commonly, infection ascends from the lower genital tract along the mucosal surface of the tube, causing an endosalpingitis. Less commonly, it may spread via the lymphatics to the wall of the tube from the uterus or other adjacent organs, causing an interstitial salpingitis. Least commonly, infection may be blood-borne. The inflammation may be non-granulomatous or granulomatous, the former being much more common.

ASCENDING INFECTION

Infection that spreads from the uterine cavity along the mucosal surface of the uterus and fallopian tube is characteristic of, for example, *Neisseria gonorrhoeae,* chlamydial infection and infection associated with the presence of an IUCD, but many cases are of a non-specific polymicrobial nature.

In an acute endosalpingitis the tube is tense and swollen, the serosa congested and the subserosal tissues oedematous. In severe infections the serosa may be covered by a fibrinous exudate. The mucosa is oedematous, hyperaemic and focally haemorrhagic. The lumen contains pus which may leak from the ostium, and the fimbria, as they become inflamed and 'sticky', tend to undergo agglutination and invagination until, finally, the ostium may be occluded. In ascending infections, as might be expected, the mucosa bears the brunt of the damage.

The oedematous tubal plicae are infiltrated by polymorphonuclear leucocytes and the lumen contains an acute inflammatory exudate and tissue debris (Figure 6.1). In severe infections, there is mucosal ulceration and the inflammatory infiltrate may extend through the wall to the peritoneum causing a local peritonitis. In repeated or chronic infections, plasma cells, lymphocytes and histiocytes predominate; the latter may, in long-standing cases, be the main cell type. If inflammation subsides rapidly or is only mild, there may be little or no residual tubal damage but unfortunately an attack of salpingitis predisposes to further

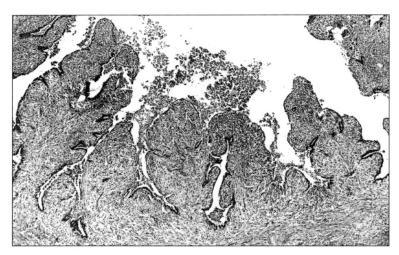

Figure 6.1 Acute endosalpingitis. The mucosal folds are oedematous and are infiltrated by acute inflammatory cells. The tube lumen contains a scanty purulent exudate.

attacks. Full recovery becomes progressively less likely with each succeeding episode, and the risk of permanent damage, leading to infertility or ectopic pregnancy, more certain.

Severe inflammation may be complicated by local or generalised peritonitis, extension of infection to the adjacent ovary, the development of a tubo-ovarian abscess or a pelvic abscess. Systemic dissemination of infection can occur, particularly in gonococcal infections, and may cause an arthritis or endocarditis. Repeated attacks of acute endosalpingitis may lead to the development of a pyosalpinx (a pus-filled fallopian tube) in which there is usually extensive ulceration of the mucosa. Such a severe degree of damage is irrecoverable.

Long-term sequelae of an endosalpingitis may be minimal and limited to minor fibrous scars in the mucosa or the musculature, or they may be major. As the ulcerated mucosa, particularly in the ampulla, heals there may be fusion of the plical folds across the lumen of the tube to produce a mesh, this being known as follicular salpingitis (Figure 6.2). Plical fusion of this type may also be seen in a tube which is, in addition, distended by clear watery fluid and in which the ostium is occluded, a condition known as a follicular hydrosalpinx. A hydrosalpinx may also occur in the absence of mucosal fold fusion and in such cases the tube assumes a retort shape and the wall is thin and translucent with the mucosa characteristically intact but rather flattened. Conversely, after prolonged or severe tubal inflammation, the

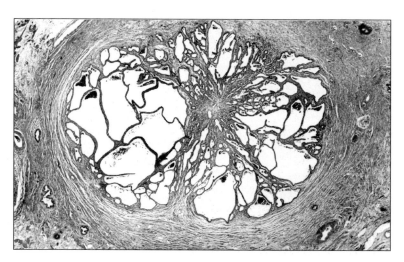

Figure 6.2 Follicular salpingitis. The plicae are extensively fused to form a honeycomb-like mesh across the tubal lumen. There is no active inflammation.

tube may be thick-walled and rather rigid as a consequence of intra-mural and subserosal fibrosis.

Changes may also occur in the isthmus as a consequence of damage, usually associated with some degree of obstruction in the outer part of the tube. Diverticula, associated with muscular hypertrophy, develop in the isthmus, a condition known as 'salpingitis isthmica nodosa' because of the nodules which can be seen or felt in the wall of the isthmus (Figure 6.3). This condition appears to be secondary to an increase in intraluminal pressure and is, in our experience, not encountered when the remainder of the tube is normal. It is not, as has been previously suggested, a direct, but rather an indirect effect of inflammation.

LYMPHATIC INFECTION

This is the form of infection which classically follows postpartum or postabortive infection and is uncommon today. The interstitial tissues of the tube are the main focus of the inflammatory assault, with rela-tive sparing of the tubal mucosa. As a consequence, the lumen may remain patent and mechanical obstruction of the tube is an unlikely outcome. However, inflammation is rarely limited to the tube wall and it is usual to find a co-existing endosalpingitis.

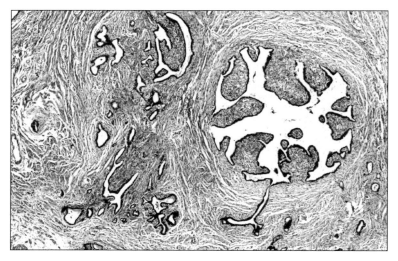

Figure 6.3 Salpingitis isthmica nodosa: diverticular disease of the fallopian tube. There are many glandular spaces within the muscle wall of the tube and, in the lower left of the field, continuity between the lumen of the tube and a diverticulum can clearly be seen.

BLOOD-BORNE INFECTION

This is typified by tuberculosis which, although it may spread directly to the tube from the peritoneal cavity, urinary tract or gastrointestinal tract, or via the lymphatics from the intestinal tract, is more likely to arise as a consequence of blood-borne infection from a distant focus.

At the time of diagnosis, the tube has often become converted into a retort-shaped, fibrotic sac which may be focally calcified and contain caseous material. Classically the tubal ostium remains patent and the fimbria relatively normal. Histological examination (Figure 6.4) shows a chronic endosalpingitis with caseating, or non-caseating, intramucosal granulomas, the latter more closely resembling sarcoid-like granulomas than the tuberculous granulomas encountered in tuberculosis elsewhere in the body. In long-standing disease the tube may be lined only by focally-calcified fibrous tissue in which it may be difficult to find specific tubercular features.

Cysts

A variety of cysts are commonly found in the tissues surrounding the fallopian tube. The majority develop in Müllerian duct remnants (paramesonephric cysts) or Wolffian duct remnants (mesonephric cysts).

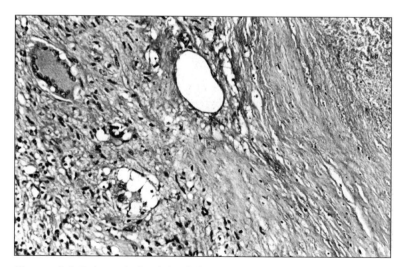

Figure 6.4 Tuberculosis of the fallopian tube. In this fibro-caseous tuberculosis the tubal lumen, to the right, is filled with caseous material and the wall, to the left, shows fibrosis and contains a Langerhans' giant cell.

Only rarely, for example when they undergo torsion or reach an unusually large size, do they become clinically apparent.

The majority of these cysts are thin-walled, often translucent and may be pedunculated. Those of Müllerian origin, which include the extremely common hydatid of Morgagni, which is pedunculated and attached to the fimbria, are lined by epithelium of tubal type. Those of Wolffian origin are lined by a single layer of cubo-columnar cells. Their walls are fibrous and those of paramesonephric origin tend to contain more muscle than do those of Müllerian origin. On rare occasions epithelial neoplasms may develop within these cysts.

The tubal serosa commonly exhibits focal transitional, or uroepithelial, metaplasia (so-called Walthard's rests) (Figure 6.5) which may also undergo cystic change. They rarely become more than a few millimetres in diameter and appear as yellow-grey specks or pinhead-size granules on the serosal surface of the tube.

Tumours of the fallopian tube

Neoplasms of the fallopian tube are rare. Carcinomas, which are the most common tumours, constitute only 0.3% of malignant gynaecological neoplasms.

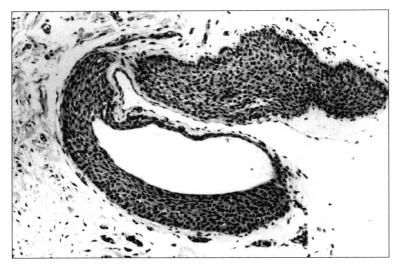

Figure 6.5 A Walthard's rest. This is on the peritoneal surface of the fallopian tube and has become cystic.

BENIGN NEOPLASMS

Benign intraluminal epithelial tumours of the tube may be sessile or polypoidal and typically form small adenofibromas. In the interstitial segment of the tube they are usually composed of endometrial tissue, whereas in the remainder of the tube they have a fibrous stroma and the epithelium is of tubal type.

Adenomatoid tumours, which are of mesothelial origin, may develop in the tubal lumen but more commonly grow eccentrically in a subserosal site, locally invaginating the tube wall. They appear as small, usually not exceeding 1–2 cm, round to ovoid, firm, grey to yellow-white, well-circumscribed nodules. Histologically (Figure 6.6), they are composed of tubules and gland-like spaces lined by a flattened cuboidal epithelium set in a fibrous stroma and they are not encapsulated.

Other very rare benign neoplasms of the fallopian tube include lipomas, which are generally subserosal, leiomyomas, fibromas, haemangiomas and neurilemmomas. Mature cystic teratomas have also, exceptionally, been described in the fallopian tube.

MALIGNANT NEOPLASMS

The commonest primary malignant neoplasms are adenocarcinomas. Most cases occur in older women, the average age being in the sixth decade of life.

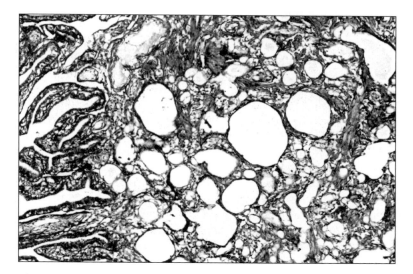

Figure 6.6 Adenomatoid tumour of the fallopian tube. Immediately deep to the tubal mucosa, to the left, there is a collection of tightly-packed small cystic spaces lying in a fine connective tissue stroma.

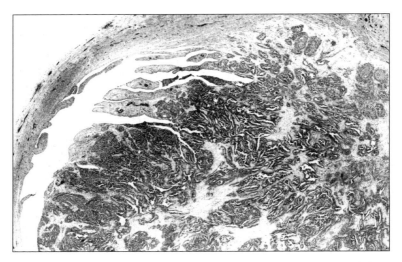

Figure 6.7 Adenocarcinoma of the fallopian tube. The lumen of the tube is distended by a polypoidal adenocarcinoma which is arising from the mucosa to the upper right.

The majority of tumours are unilateral, and between 10% and 20% are bilateral. The lesion starts as a small plaque, nodule, or polypoidal lesion within the lumen (Figure 6.7), most commonly at the junction of the middle and outer thirds of the tube, but usually by the time of diagnosis the tube is distended by tumour. The tube becomes retort-shaped and grossly resembles a hydrosalpinx or pyosalpinx but, unless there has been preceding inflammation, it is usual for the fimbria to be normal and the ostium patent. It is unusual for a tumour to have penetrated the wall of the tube.

Most carcinomas are well-differentiated papillary adenocarcinomas and closely resemble serous carcinomas of the ovary (Figure 6.8). Less well-differentiated tumours have a mixed alveolar-papillary pattern and the least well-differentiated neoplasms tend to grow in a solid fashion.

The tumour spreads directly via the tubal ostium to the peritoneum, via the uterine ostium into the uterus and directly through the tube wall to the adjacent structures. Lymphatic spread occurs to the uterus, ovary and the iliac and para-aortic lymph nodes. The average survival at five years for women with a tubal carcinoma is only about 15%.

Tubal carcinomas have to be distinguished clinically and histologically from tumours which have metastasised or spread to the tube, for example from the ovary or uterus. Such a distinction is facilitated by identifying an area of carcinoma *in situ* within the residual tubal epithelium (Figure 6.9) from which the carcinoma can be seen to arise.

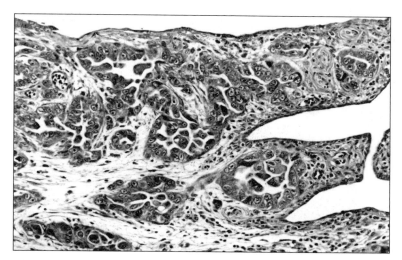

Figure 6.8 Adenocarcinoma of the fallopian tube. The mucosa is infiltrated by small neoplastic acini which are lined by pleomorphic cells of serous type.

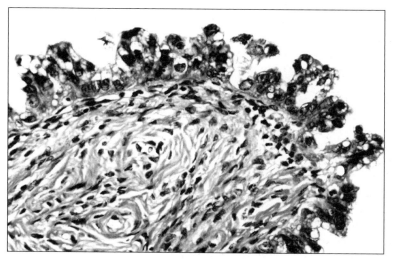

Figure 6.9 Adenocarcinoma *in situ* of the fallopian tube. The plica is covered by a stratified epithelium which is composed of cells with large pleomorphic nuclei; there is irregular papillary tufting.

7 The ovary

 Inflammation

NON-INFECTIVE INFLAMMATION

This is not common but may occur as a response to bleeding from endometriotic foci and is also seen in ovaries that have undergone torsion. A granulomatous inflammatory response may occur due to starch granules from surgical gloves, keratin derived from ruptured mature cystic teratomas, or hysterosalpingographic contrast material.

INFECTIVE INFLAMMATION

Most infections of the ovary are non-specific in nature and polymicrobial in origin. Infection may be secondary to appendicitis, diverticular disease of the colon or salpingitis and is rarely due to blood-borne infection from remote foci.

In the acute phase the ovary is reddened and oedematous. A polymorphonuclear infiltrate is present in the superficial cortex and there may be a fibrinous exudate on the ovarian surface. It is rare for infection to extend deeply into the ovary but when it does there may be abscess formation. The chronic phase is characterised by fibrosis of the ovarian surface epithelium and the formation of peri-ovarian adhesions (Figure 7.1).

Non-neoplastic cysts

Non-neoplastic cysts of the ovary may develop from the surface epithelium, follicles, endometriotic foci or may occasionally be the end result of an abscess. Most are asymptomatic, whatever their origin, but some become clinically apparent because of their large size, their undergoing torsion or their hormonal activity.

CYSTS DERIVED FROM THE SURFACE EPITHELIUM

The most common of these are the hormonally-inactive epithelial, or serous, inclusion cysts which develop as a consequence of invagination

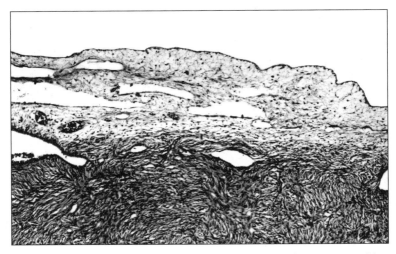

Figure 7.1 Chronic peri-oophoritis. The ovarian surface is covered by fine fibrovascular connective tissue adhesions.

of the surface epithelium of the ovary into the stroma, particularly at the site of ovulation. The invaginations lose their connection with the surface epithelium and, because of secretion of fluid, become cystic. These cysts may be single or multiple and can occur at any age. They may lie deep or superficially in the cortex and vary in size from a few millimetres to several centimetres. By convention, although perhaps illogically and incorrectly, cysts measuring more than 3cm in diameter are classed as benign serous cystadenomas. The epithelium lining the cysts is usually tubal in nature but may, less commonly, be endometrioid or endocervical in type.

CYSTS DERIVED FROM THE FOLLICLES

Follicular cysts are common but those measuring less than 2.5cm in diameter are regarded as being physiological and are classed as cystic follicles rather than as follicular cysts. Within this definition, follicular cysts are usually single, although multiple cysts of this type are encountered in the ovarian hyperstimulation and polycystic ovary syndromes.

Solitary follicular cysts can occur at any age and are thin-walled and unilocular. They range in size from 3cm to 10cm (Figure 7.2) and are lined by an inner layer of granulosa cells and an outer layer of thecal cells. Most follicular cysts are asymptomatic but some appear to be oestrogenic and are associated with symptoms such as precocious

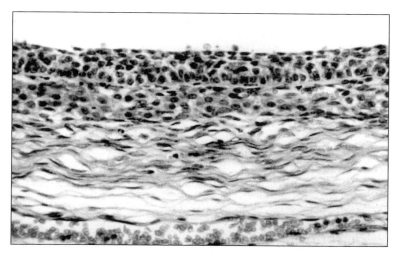

Figure 7.2 Follicular cyst of the ovary. The cyst is lined by an inner layer of granulosa cells and an outer layer of thecal cells.

puberty or menstrual disturbances and occasionally a follicular cyst may rupture and cause a haemoperitoneum. Solitary follicular cysts may develop during pregnancy and can achieve a very large size.

Corpus luteum cysts (Figure 7.3) are again distinguished from a cystic corpus luteum by their size. Cysts of this type have a convoluted lining of large luteinised granulosa cells and smaller luteinised thecal cells with an innermost layer of fibrous tissue. Such cysts probably occur when the central cavity of a ruptured follicle is unusually large or when there is excessive intrafollicular haemorrhage at the time of ovulation.

OVARIAN HYPERSTIMULATION SYNDROME

This condition is characterised by the presence of multiple theca-lutein cysts in the ovaries which are usually bilateral and may cause considerable ovarian enlargement. The cysts are of follicular origin but have a lining in which the theca interna cells are hyperplastic and heavily luteinised with granulosa cells being either absent or markedly luteinised. Cysts of this type are due to excessive stimulation of the ovary by human chorionic gonadotrophin (hCG) and may occur in:

- Normal pregnancy.
- Multiple pregnancy.
- Patients with hydatidiform mole or a choriocarcinoma.
- Women undergoing artificial stimulation of the ovary as part of the treatment of infertility.

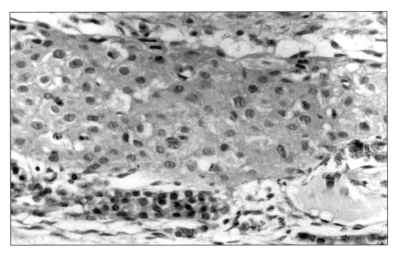

Figure 7.3 Ovarian luteal cyst.

There is an increased tendency for ovaries containing multiple theca-lutein cysts to undergo torsion and the patients may present with abdominal pain. Some patients become mildly virilised because of production of androgens by the theca-lutein cysts and ascites is occasionally encountered. The cysts usually regress after removal of their cause.

POLYCYSTIC OVARY SYNDROME (PCOS)

The term 'polycystic ovary syndrome' covers an overlapping range of disorders which have in common:

1 The presence of multiple follicular cysts in the ovaries.
2 Inappropriate gonadotrophin secretion.
3 High circulating levels of androgens.
4 Increased peripheral conversion of androgens to oestrogens.

The clinical spectrum associated with PCOS is very wide. At one extreme are asymptomatic patients whose ovarian abnormality is detected biochemically or ultrasonically only, and at the other extreme are women with infertility, obesity and hirsutism.

The typical polycystic ovary is enlarged and contains multiple follicular cysts which characteristically have a prominent outer layer of luteinised thecal cells. Other features are more variable, but there is commonly an increased amount of collagen in the superficial layers of the ovarian cortex together with stromal hyperplasia and luteinisation.

Numerous corpora fibrosa are usually present and corpora lutea are found in 30% of cases.

The pathophysiology of PCOS is complex but a constant abnormality is the presence of high, non-cyclic, levels of luteinising hormone (LH), either because of an increased pituitary sensitivity to luteinising hormone releasing factor (LHRH) or because of increased secretion of LHRH. The high LH levels stimulate theca interna cells to produce androstenedione, which is converted in the fat cells of the body into oestrone. The resulting high oestrone levels then inhibit the release of follicle-stimulating hormone (FSH). Because of the low levels of FSH, follicular growth is impaired and the granulosa cells have reduced levels of aromatase and hence a decreased ability to convert androgens to oestrogens. The elevated androgen levels in the ovary are thought to be responsible for the fibrous thickening of the superficial ovarian cortex, while the high circulating levels of the peripherally-produced oestrone increase pituitary sensitivity to LHRH and thus perpetuate the cycle. The high oestrone levels are also responsible for the development, in a proportion of these patients, of endometrial hyperplasia of simple, complex, or atypical type, which may progress to an endometrial adenocarcinoma.

Ovarian malfunction is not, however, the only factor in the hormonal disturbance of PCOS, for in some patients there is also an excess production of androstenedione by the adrenals.

Stromal hyperplasia and hyperthecosis

Stromal hyperplasia is characterised by varying degrees of non-neoplastic proliferation of ovarian stromal cells. Frequently associated with this is stromal hyperthecosis, in which there is focal luteinisation of the stromal cells.

Stromal hyperplasia results in a varying degree of diffuse or nodular ovarian enlargement, occurs most commonly in the immediately post-menopausal years, and is frequently asymptomatic. Some women, particularly those with associated hyperthecosis, show evidence of mild virilisation, or, less commonly, there may by hyperoestrogenism because of peripheral conversion of androgens to oestrone.

Massive oedema of the ovary

This term refers to a tumour-like enlargement of one or both ovaries as a result of accumulation of oedema fluid within the ovarian stroma. Massive oedema of the ovary, although quite rare, is an important and well-recognised lesion. Particularly important is its potential to present as an acute abdomen.

Affected ovaries may measure up to 25cm in diameter and when cut exude watery fluid. Histologically the oedema is diffuse but usually spares the superficial cortex.

Patients with massive oedema of the ovary are usually young and present with abdominal or pelvic pain, menstrual irregularities, or abdominal distension. Some patients are mildly virilised due to the presence of luteinised stromal cells within the oedematous ovary.

Massive oedema of the ovary is thought to result from intermittent torsion of the ovary on its pedicle with partial obstruction of venous and lymphatic drainage. In some cases the torsion appears to be secondary to a fibromatosis of the ovary.

Luteoma of pregnancy

Luteomas of pregnancy are non-neoplastic, tumour-like, solid, yellow-brown lesions of the ovary which develop from either luteinised follicular thecal cells or from luteinised non-follicular stromal cells (Figure 7.4). The luteomas may be multiple and bilateral and may be of microscopic size only or reach up to 20cm in diameter. Most pregnancy luteomas are discovered incidentally at caesarean section but a few are androgenic and associated with masculinisation of a female fetus or virilisation of the mother. Luteomas of pregnancy regress spontaneously during the postpartum period.

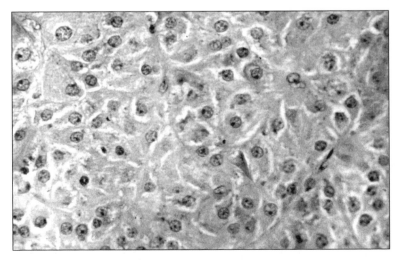

Figure 7.4 Luteoma of pregnancy.

Premature ovarian failure

This term is applied to those patients in whom there is a cessation of ovarian function before the age of 40 years.

TRUE PREMATURE MENOPAUSE

These patients have high gonadotrophin levels and small ovaries in which there is a complete absence of primordial or developing follicles, although stigmata of prior ovulation are present.

This condition is thought to be due to a primary paucity of germ cells, possibly because of inadequate migration of germ cells into the developing gonad during embryogenesis. A few cases are secondary to the use of cytotoxic drugs or radiotherapy, both of which can cause destruction of germ cells.

GONADOTROPHIN-RESISTANT OVARY SYNDROME

This syndrome may be congenital or acquired and is characterised by anovulation, low oestrogen values and high levels of gonadotrophins. The ovary contains numerous primordial follicles, sometimes showing degenerative changes, but with no evidence of follicular ripening (Figure 7.5). There is no ovarian response to the administration of exogenous gonadotrophins, even in massive doses.

This syndrome has been variously attributed to a deficiency of

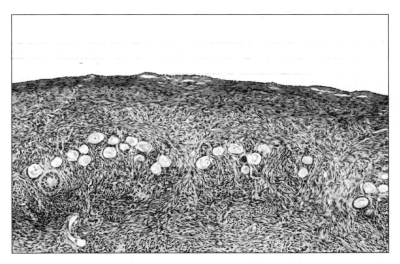

Figure 7.5 Gonadotrophin-resistant ovary. The ovarian cortex contains large numbers of primordial and primary follicles but there is no evidence of follicular maturation.

ovarian gonadotrophin receptors, the presence of antigonadotrophin receptor antibodies and to a post-receptor defect.

AUTOIMMUNE OOPHORITIS

Antibodies directed against ovarian steroid-synthesising cells are found in a proportion of women with autoimmune Addison's disease. These antibodies cross-react with steroid-synthesising cells in the adrenal glands. Patients with such antibodies present with anovulatory infertility and histologically there is a lymphocytic infiltrate around secondary or tertiary follicles.

Ovarian haemorrhage

Rupture of a corpus luteum or a corpus luteum cyst may occasionally result in bleeding into the peritoneal cavity. This occurs particularly in women receiving anticoagulant therapy.

Luteinised unruptured follicle syndrome

In this condition the follicle ripens normally but fails to release the ovum. Luteinisation of the granulosa and theca layers proceeds normally and an ovum-containing corpus luteum is formed. Hormonal activity within the ovary appears to be undisturbed, as secretory changes occur in the endometrium and thus there appears to be a primary defect in the ovum-releasing mechanism. This syndrome can be suspected if normal endometrial cyclical activity is not accompanied by ultrasonic evidence of ovulation or stigmata of ovulation on laparoscopic examination of the ovarian surface.

Tumours of the ovary

There is a huge range and variety of ovarian tumours. A simplified classification of these neoplasms defines six main groups:
1 Epithelial tumours.
2 Sex cord stromal tumours.
3 Germ cell tumours.
4 Tumours of the non-specialised tissues of the ovary.
5 Miscellaneous unclassified tumours.
6 Metastatic tumours.

(i) **EPITHELIAL TUMOURS**

These neoplasms constitute 60% of all primary ovarian tumours and 90% of those that are malignant. Most are thought to originate from undifferentiated cells in the surface, or serosal, epithelium of the ovary, either arising directly from that epithelium or from epithelial fragments which have become sequestrated into the ovarian cortex to form 'epithelial inclusion cysts'. The ovarian serosa is the direct descendant and adult equivalent of the coelomic epithelium which, during embryonic life, overlies the nephrogenital ridge and from which are derived the Müllerian ducts and the structures to which they give rise, namely the endocervical, endometrial and tubal epithelia. It is believed that undifferentiated cells in the ovarian surface epithelium retain a latent competence to differentiate along the same pathways as do their embryonic predecessors and that a neoplasm derived from these cells can, therefore, differentiate along various Müllerian pathways. Thus, those epithelial tumours differentiating along a tubal pathway constitute the serous group of neoplasms, those differentiating along endocervical lines form the mucinous tumours, and others, which pursue an endometrial course, are classed as endometrioid tumours.

The Brenner tumour also usually develops from the ovarian serosa but this type of neoplasm is formed of uro-epithelium, identical in all respects to that found in the urinary tract. Tumours of this type are therefore differentiating along Wolffian rather than Müllerian lines and it is not surprising that cells tracing their origin back to the coelomic epithelium of the nephrogenital ridge retain a residual capacity for differentiation along this line.

The final member of the group of epithelial ovarian neoplasms is the clear-cell tumour. This is identical in appearance to the clear-cell vaginal tumours that occur in DES-exposed girls and is certainly of a Müllerian nature, although admittedly not bearing a resemblance to any adult tissue of Müllerian origin. The epithelial tumours of the ovary appear to have in common, therefore, a derivation from the ovarian serosa. This unitary concept is, however, too all-embracing, for a minority of epithelial ovarian neoplasms appear to have a quite different histogenesis. Thus some mucinous tumours are formed, not of endocervical-type epithelium, but of gastrointestinal-type epithelium. Most such neoplasms probably arise from areas of gastrointestinal metaplasia within the ovarian surface epithelium, but some appear to be monophyletic teratomas. Furthermore, a proportion of both endometrioid and clear-cell neoplasms originate from pre-existing foci of ovarian endometriosis, while some Brenner tumours develop in the hilum of the ovary, possibly being derived from structures of Wolffian origin, such as the epoophoron or epigenital tubules.

Despite these exceptions, the vast majority of epithelial neoplasms are derived from the surface epithelium and each type can exist in a benign or malignant form, the various malignant tumours sharing many common characteristics and being considered collectively as 'ovarian adenocarcinoma'. In addition to the benign and malignant types of each neoplasm there exists a third form, the tumour of border-line malignancy (also known as 'tumours of low malignant potential' and as 'proliferating tumours').

(a) Serous tumours

Most benign serous neoplasms are cystic, taking the form of either a simple or papillary serous cystadenoma. Serous cystadenomas are thin-walled, usually unilocular, smooth-walled cysts, measuring from 3cm to 30cm in diameter and containing clear, straw-coloured fluid. In the papillary form of this tumour, papillae are present on one or both surfaces of the cyst. These may be few, sessile and small, or numerous, large, fleshy and pedunculated. Solid serous tumours are less common and occur either as surface serous papillomas, in which finger-like papillae project from the surface of the ovary, or as serous adeno-fibromas, which form hard, knobbly, solid masses. Serous cystade-nomas are usually lined by a single layer of flattened or cuboidal cells, but in a few instances the tubal nature of the lining epithelium may be more apparent (Figure 7.6). Certainly, the true nature of the epithe-lium is usually more overt in the papillary neoplasms, where the central core of the papillae, formed of loose fibrous tissue, is covered by an epithelium remarkably similar to that of the fallopian tube, with

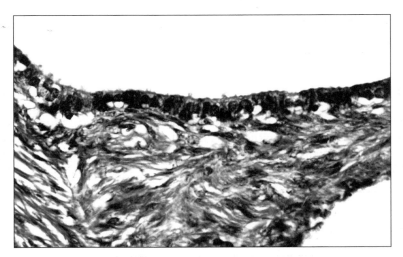

Figure 7.6 Serous cystadenoma of the ovary. The cyst is lined by a single-layered epithelium which is similar to that of the fallopian tube.

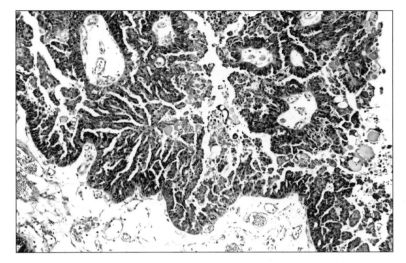

Figure 7.7 Serous adenocarcinoma of the ovary. The neoplasm is composed of papillary structures covered by an epithelium which shows extensive proliferation and budding.

secretory, ciliated, and peg cells. The serous cystadenofibroma is a predominantly fibrous tumour containing small cysts, gland-like spaces or slits lined by tubal-type epithelium.

Serous adenocarcinomas are usually large and are essentially a malignant form of the papillary serous cystadenoma, most being partially cystic and partially solid. The solid areas are formed of closely-packed or merged papillae, which often penetrate through the outer capsule of the neoplasm. Foci of necrosis or haemorrhage are common and any fluid present in the cystic portion of the tumour is commonly blood stained. Histologically, well-differentiated serous adenocarcinomas retain a papillary pattern but the epithelium shows multilayering, irregular tufting, nuclear hyperchromatism, pleomorphism and mitotic activity, whilst stromal invasion is readily apparent (Figure 7.7). From this clearly papillary form there is a spectrum of differentiation extending through to the diffuse pattern in which the tumour grows in solid sheets of cells.

Mucinous tumours

Benign mucinous tumours are almost invariably cystic, taking the form of a mucinous cystadenoma. These cystic neoplasms commonly measure between 15cm and 30cm in diameter but can attain a huge size and fill the abdominal cavity. The cysts have a thick, parchment-

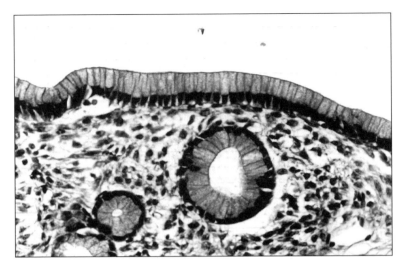

Figure 7.8 Mucinous cystadenoma of the ovary. The cyst is lined by a single layer of tall columnar, mucin-secreting epithelium: similar epithelium lines glandular acini in the cyst wall.

like wall and are usually multilocular, the locules characteristically containing clear, tenacious mucoid material. Histologically, the walls of the locules are formed of fibrous tissue and the cyst is lined by a single layer of tall, mucus-containing cells (Figure 7.8). In most tumours the epithelium is identical to that of the endocervix, but in a proportion the epithelium is of enteric type, containing goblet cells, argyrophil cells and occasionally Paneth cells.

Mucinous adenocarcinomas are usually either partially or wholly solid. Areas of necrosis or haemorrhage are common and mucoid material often exudes from their cut surface. These neoplasms show a wide spectrum of differentiation, ranging from a well-marked acinar of glandular pattern (Figure 7.9) to one in which the tumour is formed largely of solid sheets of cells in which intracellular mucus is usually present.

Mucinous tumours of any type, but usually in the benign or border-line categories, may be complicated by pseudomyxoma peritonei in which there is a marked accumulation of mucoid material in the peritoneal cavity. This has traditionally been attributed to leakage from the ovarian tumour but it has become apparent that in most, possibly all, cases there is an associated neoplasm of the appendix or, less commonly, the intestine. It has been suggested that the pseudomyxoma peritonei is secondary to the gastrointestinal lesion

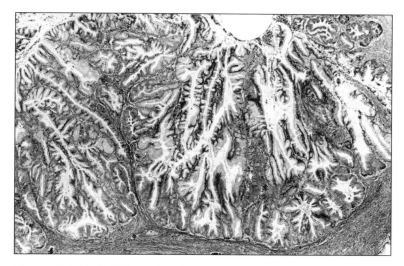

Figure 7.9 Well-differentiated mucinous adenocarcinoma of the ovary. The neoplasm consists of glandular acini lined by a mucus-secreting epithelium.

and that the apparently primary ovarian tumours in such cases are, despite their non-malignant appearance, metastases from the appendicular or intestinal neoplasm.

Endometrioid tumours

Benign endometrioid tumours appear to be very rare, although occasional examples of an endometrioid adenoma, which tends to resemble an endometrial polyp, or of an endometrioid adenofibroma, a neoplasm resembling the serous adenofibroma but in which the enclosed glands are lined by an endometrial-type epithelium, are encountered. This apparent paucity of benign endometrioid tumours may, however, be more apparent than real, for it is probable that many of the lesions classed as endometriotic cysts of the ovary are, in reality, benign endometrioid cystadenomas.

Endometrioid adenocarcinomas may be solid, partially cystic, or wholly cystic, the latter variety usually showing abundant papillary ingrowths. The defining histological feature of an endometrioid adenocarcinoma is that it mimics exactly an endometrial adenocarcinoma (Figure 7.10). Most are well differentiated and have an acinar pattern but in a minority there is a predominantly sheet-like pattern of growth. It is worth noting that any neoplasm which occurs in the endometrium can also arise in the ovary as a variant of an

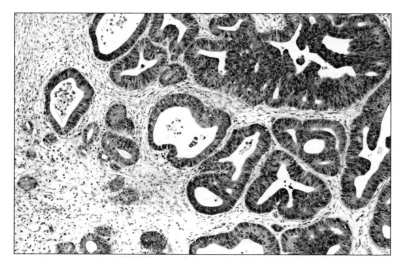

Figure 7.10 Well-differentiated endometrioid adenocarcinoma of the ovary. The tumour is similar in appearance to an adenocarcinoma of the endometrium.

endometrioid adenocarcinoma and thus carcinosarcomas, adenosarcomas and endometrial stromal sarcomas can all occur in the ovary as forms of endometrioid neoplasia.

Brenner tumours

The majority of Brenner tumours are benign and occur as small, solid, well-circumscribed nodules with a smooth or bosselated surface and a hard, whorled, greyish-white, cut surface. Histologically, the Brenner tumour is characterised by well-demarcated nests and branching columns of epithelial cells set in a fibrous stroma (Figure 7.11). The epithelial nests are formed of round or polygonal cells with distinct limiting membranes, abundant cytoplasm and ovoid or round nuclei which are often prominently grooved. Cystic change in the centre of the cell nests is common and these cystic spaces may be lined by flattened, cuboidal or columnar cells.

Malignant Brenner tumours may resemble architecturally a benign Brenner neoplasm but show a marked overgrowth of the epithelial component with nuclear hyperchromatism, cytological atypia, mitotic activity and stromal invasion. Some malignant Brenner tumours develop, however, as pure transitional cell carcinomas (Figure 7.12), identical in all respects to their counterparts in the urinary tract.

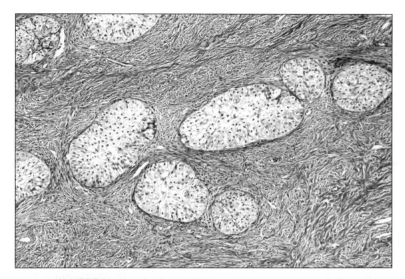

Figure 7.11 Brenner tumour of the ovary. The neoplasm is formed of highly atypical infiltrating transitional epithelium.

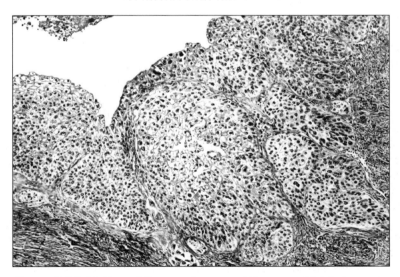

Figure 7.12 Malignant Brenner tumour of the ovary. This is formed of highly atypical infiltrating transitional epithelium.

Clear-cell tumours

Benign clear-cell neoplasms are distinctly uncommon and take the form of clear-cell adenofibromas in which gland-like spaces set in fibrous tissue are lined by cells with clear cytoplasm and hobnail nuclei.

Most clear-cell tumours are adenocarcinomas. These are usually large and only a minority are solid, most being cystic with solid areas. The solid areas tend to be soft and fleshy whereas the cystic portions are commonly multilocular and often contain mucoid material. These neoplasms have a complex histological appearance, showing an admixture of papillary, cystic, glandular and solid growth forms (Figure 7.13). The cysts and acini tend to be lined by cells with clear cytoplasm and large, deeply-staining nuclei which protrude into the lumen (hobnail nuclei).

Ovarian adenocarcinoma

The malignant forms of the various epithelial tumours of the ovary are, in clinical practice, usually grouped together into the single entity of ovarian adenocarcinoma.

Serous and endometrioid tumours form the bulk of ovarian adenocarcinoma, mucinous tumours are less common and clear-cell carcinoma and malignant Brenner tumours are relatively rare.

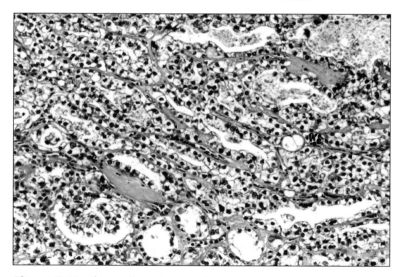

Figure 7.13 Clear cell carcinoma of the ovary. This is formed of highly atypical infiltrating transitional epithelium.

It has been widely believed that tumour type is of some prognostic significance with, for example, serous adenocarcinomas pursuing a more malignant course than do their endometrioid counterparts. Multivariate analysis has, however, shown this not to be true. The only two significant prognostic factors are the clinical stage at the time of diagnosis and the histological grade of the neoplasm.

Staging of ovarian adenocarcinomas is dependent upon a knowledge of their mode of spread. Local spread is by direct seeding on to the peritoneum with implantation of secondary deposits in the contralateral ovary, the pouch of Douglas, the omentum and on the surface of the uterus. Malignant cells are also seeded into the small amount of fluid that is normally present in the peritoneal cavity. This fluid tends to circulate upwards along the paracolic gutters and, whereas on the left side the circulation of the fluid is dammed by the phrenico-colic ligament, there is no such bar on the right side of the abdomen and the fluid reaches the under surface of the right leaf of the diaphragm. Tumour cells are thus carried into the para-colic gutters and to the right leaf of the diaphragm, these being sites of early metastasis. Lymphatic spread is to the pelvic nodes. Spread to the para-aortic nodes also occurs, at a relatively early stage in the growth of the tumour. Blood-borne spread is a late and uncommon event and is usually to the liver and lungs.

Currently, ovarian adenocarcinoma has a gloomy prognosis, the overall five-year survival rate being only in the region of 25–30%. Unfortunately, little is known of the aetiology of this lethal form of neoplasia. It has been suggested that the ground is prepared for eventual neoplastic change in the surface epithelium by the repetitive minor trauma of ovulation, a view lent credence by the finding that both oral contraception and pregnancy, each associated with inhibition of ovulation, decrease the risk of developing ovarian adenocarcinoma. The protective effect of pregnancy is cumulative but, nevertheless, simple inhibition of ovulation is not the entire explanation for these effects, for one pregnancy offers the same degree of protection as does three years' use of oral contraceptives.

Genetic factors are also important and about five percent of ovarian cancers develop in women with 'ovarian cancer genes' such as the BRCA-1 and BRCA-2 genes.

Epithelial tumours of borderline malignancy

These neoplasms, also known as 'tumours of low malignant potential' or 'proliferative tumours', lie in the grey area between clearly benign and overtly malignant epithelial ovarian neoplasms. It is largely the serous and mucinous borderline tumours which have been clearly

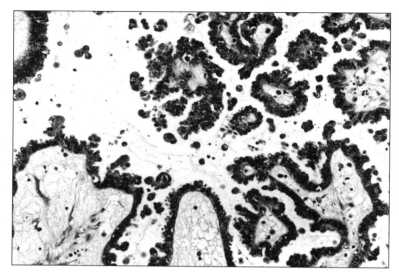

Figure 7.14 A serous papillary tumour of borderline malignancy. The papillae are covered by cells which are multilayered, rather pleomorphic and show irregular budding. There is no stromal invasion.

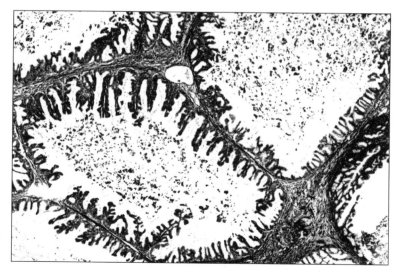

Figure 7.15 A mucinous tumour of borderline malignancy. The neoplastic locules are lined by columnar, mucin-secreting cells which form tufts and irregular papillae. There is no stromal invasion.

defined, with borderline endometrioid, Brenner and clear-cell neoplasms forming a more controversial group. Borderline mucinous and serous tumours are relatively common and macroscopically closely resemble their fully benign counterparts. Histologically (Figures 7.14 and 7.15), the epithelial component of these neoplasms shows some, or indeed all, of the characteristics of malignancy, such as multi-layering, irregular budding, cytological atypia, nuclear hyperchromatism and pleomorphism, and mitotic activity. There is, however, no stromal invasion and this lack of invasiveness is both a defining feature of these neoplasms and an indication of their unique biological status. The tumours, particularly those of serous type, may show a homogeneously borderline pattern throughout, or there may be an admixture, within a single neoplasm, of clearly benign epithelium and of epithelium showing borderline characteristics. It must be stressed that the diagnosis of a tumour of borderline malignancy is a positive one that is based on the histological findings and that the use of this term is not indicative of any indecision on the pathologist's part as to whether the tumour is benign or malignant.

In a proportion of borderline tumours, particularly and perhaps only those of serous type, there appears to be extraovarian spread with multiple small tumour nodules dotted around on the peritoneum and omentum. Some of these are possibly seedling implants from neoplasms with an exophytic growth pattern but most are not true metastases, developing *in situ* within the submesothelial connective tissues (the secondary Müllerian system). Histologically, these may show a fully benign pattern (endosalpingiosis), a pattern resembling that seen in a borderline tumour (atypical endosalpingiosis), or can appear invasive and resemble true metastases from an adenocarcinoma. It is currently not clear whether these histological findings are of prognostic significance. If peritoneal lesions do progress they do so in an indolent fashion. Tumours of borderline malignancy without extra-ovarian lesions have an excellent prognosis.

SEX CORD STROMAL TUMOURS

The neoplasms contain granulosa cells, Sertoli cells, thecal cells, Leydig cells, fibroblasts of specialised stromal origin, or the precursors of these cells, either singly or in any combination. It has been thought that all these cells are ultimately derived from the mesenchyme of the genital ridge but it is more likely that both granulosa and Sertoli cells differentiate from the sex cords of the developing gonad. These cords probably originate from the coelomic epithelium rather than from mesenchyme. It is believed that sex cord cells can, depending on the nature of the developing gonad, differentiate into either Sertoli or granulosa cells, and that this bisexual potentiality is retained in undifferentiated sex cord cells in the adult gonad, granulosa cell tumours and Sertoli cell neoplasms thus being homologous with each other. Neoplasia of these cells is often accompanied by a reactive stromal proliferation which, in the case of a granulosa cell tumour, often shows thecomatous differentiation and in Sertoli cell neoplasms shows Leydig cell differentiation. Pure stromal neoplasms, thecomas and Leydig cell tumours can also occur.

(a) ## Granulosa cell tumours – adult type

3-5% of all ovarian ca.
70% of sex cord stromal tumours

These are usually solid neoplasms which may be hard or rubbery, their cut surface is white, yellow or grey and their average size is about 12cm in diameter. A proportion of granulosa cell neoplasms are, however, partially cystic and a few are wholly cystic, resembling a cystadenoma.

Histologically, the cells in a granulosa cell tumour are small, round or polygonal, having little cytoplasm and indistinct cell boundaries (Figure 7.16). Their large, round or ovoid pale nuclei characteristically show longitudinal grooving. The cells are arranged in a variety of patterns and although in any individual neoplasm a particular pattern may predominate, there is usually an admixture of cellular arrange-

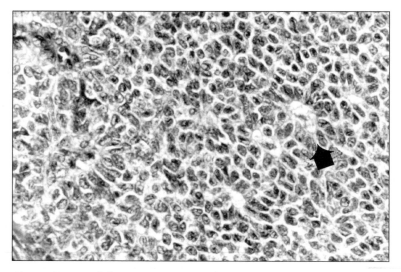

Figure 7.16 Adult-type granulosa cell tumour of the ovary. The solid neoplasm is composed of uniform oval cells with regular dark staining of nuclei which are grooved. Call–Exner bodies are present (arrowed).

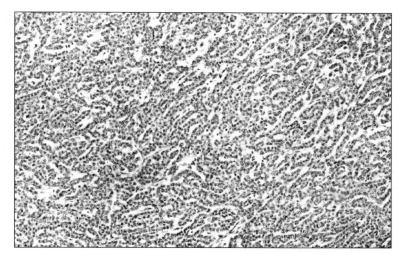

Figure 7.17 Adult type granulosa cell tumour of the ovary. The cells are arranged in a fine trabecular pattern.

ments. In the insular pattern the cells are arranged in compact masses or islands whereas in the trabecular pattern the cells form anastomosing ribbons or cords (Figure 7.17). Alternatively, the cells may be arranged in sheets to give a diffuse pattern. In the multifollicular pattern, granulosa cells are arranged around small spaces containing nuclear fragments, these being the Call–Exner bodies, whilst a macrofollicular pattern is due to liquefaction within islands of granulosa cells. In cystic granulosa cell tumours the cyst lining resembles that of a Graafian follicle but usually contains microfollicles.

A granulosa cell tumour may produce non-specific pelvic tumour symptoms, but about 75% of patients with such neoplasms have symptoms indicative of oestrogen secretion by the neoplasm. Thus, in young girls these tumours commonly result in isosexual precocious pseudopuberty, whereas in women of reproductive age complaints of irregular menstruation or menorrhagia are common. In postmenopausal patients granulosa cell tumours cause postmenopausal vaginal bleeding and sometimes a resurgence of libido. Endometrial changes, such as simple or atypical hyperplasia, are commonly found in association with granulosa cell tumours whilst an endometrial adenocarcinoma occurs in six to ten percent of cases. A few granulosa cell tumours, particularly those which are cystic, appear to be androgenic rather than oestrogenic.

All granulosa cell tumours should be considered as potentially malignant, although the degree of malignancy is often very low and

granulosa cell tumours tend to be confined to the ovary & potentially slow growing tumour   secrete E2 + inhibin the course pursued by the tumour is frequently very indolent. Recurrence or metastases tend to occur late, commonly after five years, not infrequently after ten years and sometimes after 20 years. The histological pattern of the tumour is of no prognostic importance; indeed it is doubtful if there are any prognostic indicators apart from extraovarian spread. The long-term survival rate for patients with this neoplasm is between 50% and 60%.

(b) Juvenile granulosa cell tumour

This is a histological variant of granulosa cell tumour which occurs predominantly in patients aged less than 20 years, although some neoplasms of this type arise in older women. The tumours (Figure 7.18) contain follicles and cysts lined by granulosa cells, together with solid areas showing a haphazard admixture of granulosa and thecal cells which can show a striking degree of luteinisation. The neoplastic cells lack the nuclear grooving characteristic of an adult-type granulosa cell tumour and there is often a moderate degree of cytological atypia and mitotic activity.

About five percent of juvenile granulosa cell tumours behave in a malignant fashion and tend to recur rapidly and disseminate widely throughout the abdominal cavity within two years of the initial diagnosis, a pattern of malignant behaviour quite unlike that of an adult-type granulosa cell tumour.

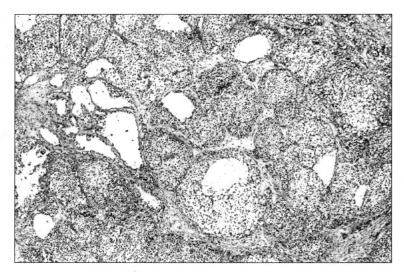

Figure 7.18 Juvenile granulosa cell tumour of the ovary. Numerous macrofollicles are present.

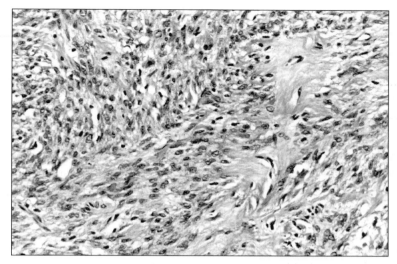

Figure 7.19 Fibrothecoma of the ovary. The tumour cells are spindle or oval shaped.

Thecomas (fibrothecoma)

These are solid tumours which are formed of plump, pale, ovoid, or spindle-shaped cells with indistinct borders which are arranged in interlacing bundles or anastomosing trabeculae (Figure 7.19). These neoplasms arise from the ovarian mesenchyme and occur most commonly in postmenopausal women. They are oestrogenic and produce symptoms similar to those noted in patients with granulosa cell tumours. Some thecomas show focal luteinisation and such neoplasms may be weakly androgenic.

Thecomas are, with rare exceptions, benign. Malignant thecomas are not distinguishable from fibrosarcomas.

Fibromas

Neoplasms of this type probably arise from ovarian gonadal stroma. They are similar to fibromas elsewhere in the body, but it is of note that a proportion of ovarian fibromas are, for unknown reasons, accompanied by ascites and a hydrothorax (Meig's syndrome). Ovarian fibromas also tend to occur in association with the basal cell naevus, or Gorlin's syndrome, under which unusual circumstances the tumours tend to be bilateral, multifocal and calcified.

Fibromas are benign but a few show increased cellularity, pleomorphism and mitotic activity. Tumours showing these features to only a mild degree are classed as cellular fibromas which will recur if incompletely removed, and those with more marked atypia and mitotic activity are classed as fibrosarcomas, highly aggressive neoplasms with a poor prognosis.

(e) **Androblastoma**

Androblastomas are neoplasms composed of Sertoli cells, Leydig cells or a combination of the two cell types.

(i) Pure Sertoli cell neoplasms are rare and occur as small, solid, yellowish masses. Histologically (Figure 7.20) the tumours show highly-differentiated tubules lined by a single layer of radically-orientated Sertoli cells which commonly contain lipid droplets and are occasionally distended and vacuolated by fat. Sertoli cell neoplasms are, with very rare exceptions, benign, and about 50% appear to be oestrogenic, the remainder lacking any obvious endocrinological activity.

(ii) Leydig cell neoplasms may arise either from stromal cells or from pre-existing hilar cells. The tumours are small, yellowish-brown and consist of Leydig cells arranged in sheets or solid cords (Figure 7.21). The cytoplasm of the Leydig cells is markedly eosinophilic and their nuclei are large and centrally placed. Reinke's crystals, slender rod-shaped bodies with rounded, tapering, or square ends, are present in about 50% of these neoplasms but are irregularly distributed and often difficult to detect.

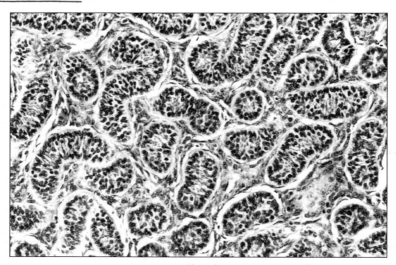

Figure 7.20 Sertoli cell tumour of the ovary. The neoplasm is composed of narrow tubules lined by cubo-columnar cells set in a fibrous stroma.

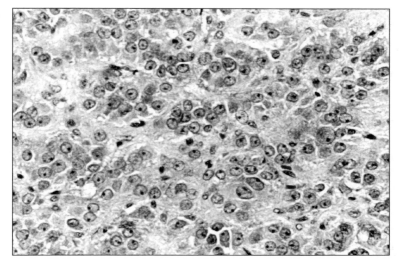

Figure 7.21 Leydig cell tumour of the ovary. The tumour cells are uniform in shape and size but the nuclei are grouped and irregularly dispersed.

Leydig cell tumours are nearly always virilising, although occasional oestrogenic or endocrinologically inert examples are encoutered. The vast majority (95%) are benign but exceptional tumours of this type give rise to metastases, a possibility not predictable on any histological grounds.

(fu) Sertoli–Leydig cell tumours are generally solid neoplasms which show a wide range of histological differentiation. Well-differentiated neoplasms are formed of tubules lined by Sertoli cells with variable numbers of Leydig cells between the tubules. In less well-differentiated tumours the Sertoli cells are arranged in cords, solid tubules, or trabeculae (Figure 7.22), these being set in a mesenchymal stroma containing clusters or nodules of Leydig cells. Poorly-differentiated Sertoli–Leydig neoplasms (Figure 7.23) consist largely of sheets of spindle-shaped cells in which occasional irregular cord-like structures or imperfectly-formed tubules may be recognised with Leydig cells also present in small clusters.

Sertoli–Leydig cell neoplasms can occur at any age but the majority develop in women aged between 10 and 35 years. These tumours are usually androgenic and produce virilisation. The well-differentiated neoplasms always behave in a benign fashion but between 10% and 40% of the less well-differentiated tumours behave in a malignant fashion, this being particularly the case for the poorly-differentiated tumours.

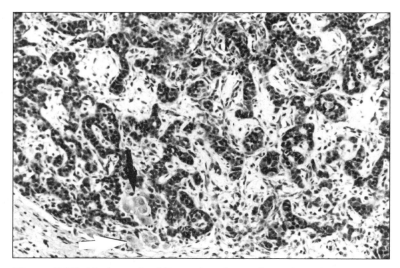

Figure 7.22 Moderately-differentiated Sertoli-Leydig cell tumour of the ovary. The neoplasm is composed of cords of darkly staining cells, resembling sex cords, set in a fibrous stroma in which there are small numbers of Leydig cells (arrowed) with pale-staining cytoplasm.

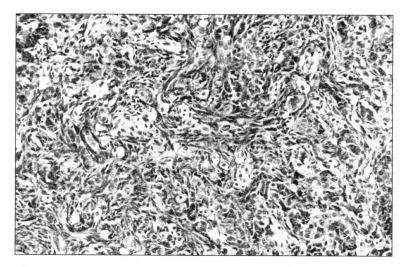

Figure 7.23 Poorly-differentiated Sertoli-Leydig cell tumour of the ovary. The neoplasm consists of bundles of spindle cells admixed with Leydig cells.

Recurrence or metastases, characteristically to the omentum, abdominal lymph nodes or liver, are usually apparent within one year of initial diagnosis.

Gynandroblastoma

A true gynandroblastoma contains an admixture of areas showing unequivocal granulosa cell differentiation and of other areas in which there is equally incontrovertible Sertoli cell differentiation. Such tumours are extremely rare, consequently their pattern of behaviour is still largely undetermined.

Sex cord tumour with annular tubules

This uncommon, but histologically distinctive, tumour contains rounded nests in which epithelial-like cells surround hyaline bodies (Figure 7.24). The epithelial-like cells, which are thought to be immature sex cord cells, are palisaded along the periphery of the cell nests and around the hyaline bodies. About one-third of these tumours are associated with the Peutz–Jeghers syndrome and in such circumstances the lesions are usually bilateral, of microscopic size, calcified and benign. The tumours not associated with the Peutz–Jeghers syndrome are unilateral, large, uncalcified, often show an overgrowth of either granulosa or Sertoli cells and behave in a malignant fashion in about 20% of cases.

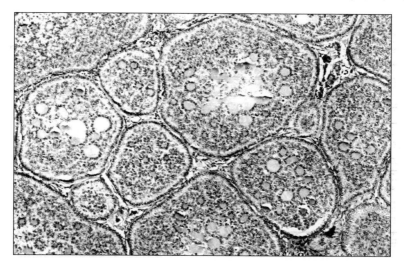

Figure 7.24 Sex cord tumour with annular tubules. The neoplasm is composed of discrete islands of immature sex cord cells palisaded around amorphous proteinaceous material.

(3) **GERM CELL TUMOURS**

Tumours derived from germ cells may show no evidence of differentiation into either embryonic or extra-embryonic tissues, can differentiate into embryonic tissue, or may differentiate along extra-embryonic pathways into trophoblast or yolk sac structures.

Very little is known about the aetiology of germ cell neoplasms. Extensive studies of naturally-occurring gonadal teratomas in highly inbred genetic strains of mice and of experimentally-induced murine teratomas have, however, indicated that teratomas arise from pathogenetic pregnancies (that is, in which there has been no fertilisation of the ovum) which undergo a short period of embryogenesis and then break up to yield a neoplasm. Genetic studies of human ovarian teratomas strongly suggest that these tumours arise in a similar manner.

Dysgerminoma (non embryonic or poschembryonic)

This neoplasm is formed of cells which closely resemble primordial germ cells, showing no evidence of differentiation into either embryonic or extra-embryonic structures. As such the tumour is identical to the seminoma of the testis.

Dysgerminomas commonly arise in patients aged between 10 and 30 years. Their development is usually announced by non-specific tumour symptoms, although isosexual precocious pseudopuberty is sometimes seen in young girls. These neoplasms have a particular tendency to arise in patients with developmental abnormalities of the gonads, although the vast majority of dysgerminomas occur in otherwise fully normal individuals. + eg Androgen insealing /syes

The tumours are solid and usually measure about 12cm in diameter. Histologically (Figure 7.25), the neoplastic cells are large, uniform, round, oval or polyhedral, with well-defined limiting membranes, abundant cytoplasm and large vesicular nuclei. The cells are commonly arranged in solid nests separated by delicate fibrous septa but may form cords or strands embedded in a fibrous stroma. A lymphocytic infiltration of the stroma, sometimes aggregated into follicles with germinal centres and small stromal granulomas, are characteristic features.

Dysgerminomas are malignant. Rupture of their enveloping 'capsule' often leads to direct implantation of tumour onto the pelvic peritoneum and omentum and lymphatic spread occurs relatively early to the para-aortic, retroperitoneal, mediastinal and supraclavicular nodes. Haematogenous spread to the liver, lungs, kidneys and bone occurs at a late stage. These tumours are, however, highly sensitive to both radiation and chemotherapy and the five-year survival rate is well over 90%.

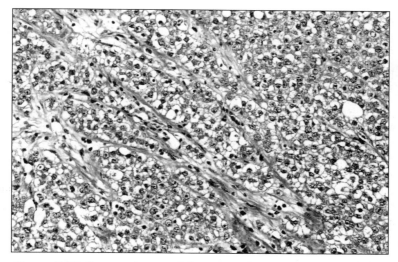

Figure 7.25 Dysgerminoma of the ovary. The neoplasm is composed of undifferentiated germ cells with vesicular nuclei and clear cytoplasm. These are arranged in cords, trabeculae and islands: there is a scattering of lymphocytes between the tumour cords.

Choriocarcinomas - Eoche embyaic

These are germ cell tumours showing trophoblastic differentiation. They are often combined with other malignant germ cell elements but pure ovarian choriocarcinomas are occasionally encountered. In women of reproductive age it is usually impossible to tell whether such a neoplasm is a germ cell tumour, a metastasis from a uterine choriocarcinoma or a tumour arising from the placental tissue of an ectopic ovarian pregnancy. In premenarchal and postmenopausal patients this problem does not arise and here an origin from ovarian germ cells can be readily accepted. The histological appearances of such tumours are identical to those of gestational uterine choriocarcinomas. Nevertheless, ovarian choriocarcinomas respond poorly to the chemotherapeutic regime which is so successful for uterine gestational choriocarcinomas.

Yolk sac tumours - Eoche embyaic

These rare neoplasms, also known as endodermal sinus tumours, represent neoplastic germ cell differentiation along extra-embryonic lines into mesoblast and yolk sac endoderm. They share with yolk sac structures the ability to secrete alpha-fetoprotein (AFP).

Yolk sac tumours form large masses showing conspicuous haemorrhage, necrosis and microcystic change. Their histological appearances

Also secrete d₁ Antitrypsn

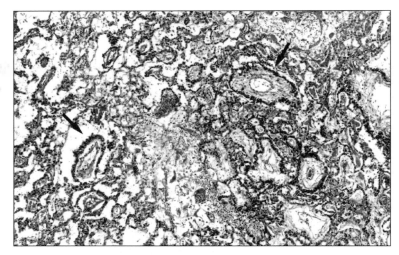

Figure 7.26 Yolk sac tumour of the ovary. In this field there are several Schiller-Duval bodies (arrowed): elsewhere the neoplasm forms a delicate reticular mesh and small cystic structures.

are very complex (Figure 7.26) but there is characteristically a loose, vacuolate labyrinthine network containing microcysts lined by flattened cells together with Schiller–Duval bodies which have a mesenchymal core containing a central capillary and an epithelial investment of cuboidal or columnar cells. A glandular pattern is often seen and there may be hepatoid or endodermal differentiation. Eosinophilic hyaline droplets are present in nearly all yolk sac tumours and these consist predominantly of AFP.

Yolk sac tumours occur most commonly in girls aged between four and 20 years, present solely with non-specific tumour symptoms and are highly aggressive neoplasms which spread rapidly within the abdomen and to distant sites. Their previously appalling prognosis has been much improved by the introduction of effective chemotherapy and the prognosis is now relatively hopeful in a substantial proportion of cases. The progress of the tumour, its response to chemotherapy and the development of recurrence can all be monitored by serial estimations of serum AFP levels.

Teratomas

These are germ cell neoplasms showing differentiation along embryonic lines. In most there is a melange of tissues but in some, known as monophyletic teratomas, there is differentiation along only a single tissue pathway, for example solely into thyroid tissue. The terms 'benign' and 'malignant' are not truly applicable to teratomas, for the prognosis of any individual neoplasm is determined not by the usual criteria of malignancy but by the degree of maturity of its constituent tissues. Those in which all the components are fully mature behave in a benign fashion and increasing degrees of tissue immaturity are associated with a progressive tendency towards the neoplasm running a malignant course. Hence teratomas are classed as either 'immature' or 'mature', the term 'malignant' being reserved for those cases in which true malignant change has occurred in a mature teratoma, such as when a squamous cell carcinoma develops in a mature cystic teratoma.

The vast majority of ovarian teratomas are mature and cystic. Such neoplasms, often known as 'dermoids', account for between 10% and 20% of all ovarian tumours and for 97% of ovarian teratomas, these being usually cystic. Just over ten percent of mature cystic teratomas are bilateral, most measure between 5cm and 15cm in diameter and some are pedunculated. They are round or ovoid with a smooth or slightly wrinkled outer surface. On opening, the teratomas are usually unilocular and have a smooth or granular inner surface. There is commonly a focal hillock-like protuberance into the cyst lumen, this being usually known as Rokitansky's tubercle or the mamillary body. The cysts nearly always contain greasy sebaceous material and hair. Teeth are present in about a third and may lie loose in the cyst, be embedded in the wall or attached to a rudimentary jaw bone. Histologically, the cyst is almost invariably lined by squamous epithe-

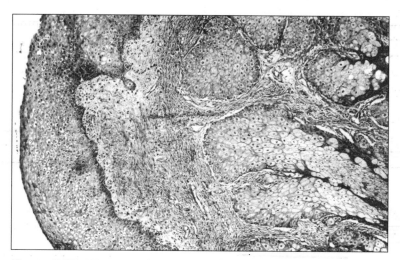

Figure 7.27 Mature cystic teratoma of the ovary. The cyst is lined by mature squamous epithelium and the wall contains sebaceous glands.

lium and skin appendages are also very common (Figure 7.27). Fat, respiratory-type epithelium, bone, cartilage, neural tissue, gastrointestinal-type epithelium, thyroid and salivary gland tissue are frequent components. Breast or pituitary tissue is uncommonly encountered and some tissues, such as kidney, pancreas and spleen, are noticeable for their almost complete absence. There is currently no explanation for this apparent selectivity.

Ninety per cent of mature cystic teratomas are found in women of reproductive age and most are asymptomatic incidental findings. However, some patients suffer complications such as torsion or rupture, both of which present as an acute abdominal emergency. Sometimes a rupture is less acute and slow leakage of cyst contents produces a chronic chemical peritonitis. Occasionally patients present with a haemolytic anaemia due, it is believed, to the presence of tumour antigens which evoke antibodies that cross-react with erythrocytic antigens.

True malignant change occurs in between one percent and two percent of patients with mature cystic teratomas, this usually taking the form of a squamous cell carcinoma.

A small proportion of mature teratomas are solid rather than cystic but most solid teratomas are of the immature variety. These are rare neoplasms which occur principally during the first two decades of life. Microscopic examination of such neoplasms reveals an admixture of both mature and immature tissues, although immature mesenchyme or neuro-epithelium (Figure 7.28) tend to be dominant features. Immature teratomas behave in a malignant fashion, implanting on to pelvic peritoneum, metastasising to retroperitoneal and para-aortic lymph nodes, and being disseminated via the bloodstream to the lungs and liver. The previously extremely poor prognosis of these neoplasms has been transformed by chemotherapy, with approximately 60% of patients now surviving.

Monophyletic teratomas, in which differentiation is into only one tissue, are characterised by the struma ovarii which consists solely or predominantly of tissue that is histologically, physiologically and pharmacologically identical to that of the normal cervical thyroid gland (Figure 7.29). This ovarian thyroid tissue may function autonomously to produce a 'pelvic' hyperthyroidism, can show the changes of a lymphocytic thyroiditis and sometimes undergoes malignant change with a resulting thyroid adenocarcinoma which can metastasise to lymph nodes, liver and lungs.

Many carcinoid tumours of the ovary occur in a mature cystic teratoma, in association with gastrointestinal- or respiratory-type epithelium, but a few are pure and not admixed with any other tissues,

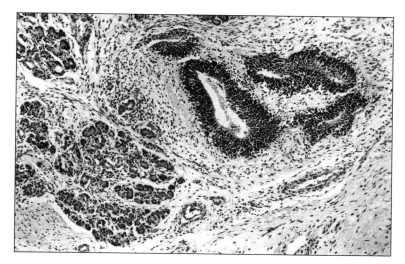

Figure 7.28 Immature teratoma of the ovary. To the right of the field there are rosette-like structures: these are immature neuro-epithelial tissue. To the left there are immature glandular structures.

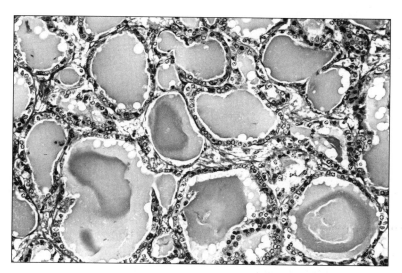

Figure 7.29 Struma ovarii. The neoplasm is composed of mature thyroid tissue.

* All Solid teratomes are neb immature
immature teratome leads to be unilotec

these being regarded as monophyletic teratomas. Ovarian carcinoid tumours are similar to those that occur in the gastrointestinal tract, usually showing either an insular or a trabecular pattern (Figure 7.30), but are associated with a high incidence of a typical carcinoid syndrome, this reflecting the ability of these tumours to secrete products directly into the systemic, rather than the portal, circulation.

A strumal carcinoid is a rare neoplasm that combines the features of a struma ovarii and a carcinoid tumour. It is thought that the carcinoid component of these neoplasms is derived from the parafollicular cells and that it is thus homologous with the medullary carcinoma of the thyroid gland.

4 TUMOURS OF NON-SPECIALISED OVARIAN TISSUE

The only common ovarian tumours of this type are fibromas (see pages 109–110).

5 MISCELLANEOUS TUMOURS

Steroid cell tumours

These are neoplasms which have an endocrine-type architecture and are formed of cells which resemble adrenocortical cells, Leydig cells, or luteinised stromal cells. All are thought to derive from the ovarian

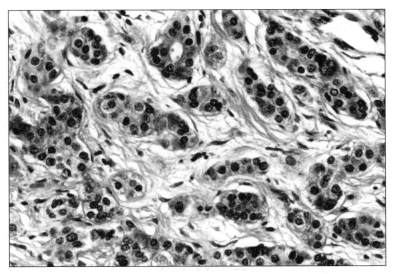

Figure 7.30 Carcinoid tumour of the ovary. Uniform cells with round nuclei form trabeculae between which there is fibrous tissue.

stroma and may be accompanied by evidence of virilisation. Some of the adrenal-like tumours are associated with clinical features suggestive of Cushing's syndrome (Figure 7.31).

Small-cell carcinoma

Two types of small-cell carcinoma occur in the ovary, both being of unknown origin and nature. Small-cell carcinomas with hypercalcaemia are rapidly-growing, highly-aggressive neoplasms which occur in young women and hypercalcaemia is present in about 50% of cases. These tumours are formed of sheets of small cells, often admixed with larger cells, which show areas of cavitation, haemorrhage and necrosis. The other type of small-cell carcinoma is not associated with hypercalcaemia, occurs in women of menopausal age, can be bilateral and histologically resembles a small-cell carcinoma of the bronchus.

METASTATIC TUMOURS OF THE OVARY

The ovary is a common site of metastasis, particularly from primary sites in the breast, gastrointestinal tract and uterus. Thus, ovarian metastases are found in approximately one-third of women dying of malignant disease, and between 10% and 20% of ovarian tumours which appear originally to be primary to that site eventually turn out to be metastatic in nature.

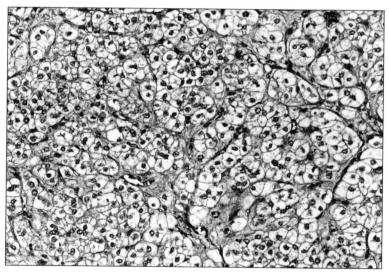

Figure 7.31 Steroid cell tumour of the ovary which has an adrenal-like appearance.

Ovarian metastases are often bilateral and commonly show extensive areas of haemorrhage and necrosis. Histologically there tends to be a multinodular pattern and the metastases usually reiterate the appearances of the primary tumour.

A particular form of metastatic ovarian neoplasm is the Krukenberg tumour. These neoplasms are usually bilateral and solid. The metastatic carcinoma cells occur singly, in clumps or sheets, or may form tubules and a proportion are mucus-containing and have their nuclei displaced laterally to give a 'signet-ring' appearance (Figure 7.32). The non-neoplastic stromal cells show a degree of pleomorphism and mitotic activity and are often incorrectly described as having a pseudosarcomatous appearance. Krukenberg tumours are usually metastases from either gastric or colonic carcinomas and the view that gastric carcinomas metastasise to the ovaries by transcoelomic spread is now giving way to the belief that such tumours spread to the ovary via the lymphatics.

Endometriosis

Endometriosis is the presence of ectopic endometrial tissue in an extrauterine location. The ectopic tissue occurs most frequently in the ovaries, pouch of Douglas, uterine ligaments, pelvic peritoneum, recto-

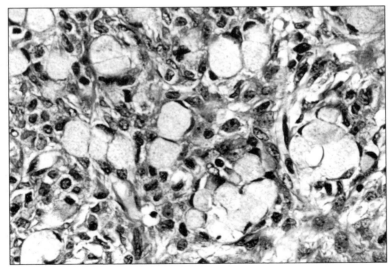

Figure 7.32 Krukenberg tumour of the ovary. The fibrous ovarian stroma is infiltrated by single cells and cell clusters with eccentric nuclei and vacuolated cytoplasm (signet-ring cells).

vaginal septum, cervix, appendix, inguinal hernial sacs and the bowel. Foci of endometriosis are occasionally encountered in surgical scars, the vulva, the bladder, the skin or at the umbilicus, and exceptional instances of lesions occurring in lymph nodes, kidneys, limbs, pleura and lungs have been recorded.

The pathogenesis of endometriosis is still uncertain but one probable mechanism for its development is the reflux of endometrial tissue through the fallopian tubes as a result of retrograde menstruation, with subsequent implantation on, and growth in, the ovaries, pelvic peritoneum and uterine ligaments.

An alternative, but not mutually exclusive, view is that, in the pelvis at least, endometriosis arises as a result of endometrial metaplasia of the peritoneal serosa. This is a feasible hypothesis and it may well be that such metaplasia is induced by contact with regurgitated fragments of endometrium which, after initiating the metaplastic process, subsequently die and are absorbed. The existence of endometriotic foci in lymph nodes and in distant sites, such as the lung, can clearly not be explained by this mechanism and hence lymphatic or haematogenous dissemination of endometrium must be evoked in such cases. It is almost certain that there is no single pathogenetic mechanism that applies to all cases of endometriosis.

If, however, retrograde menstruation occurs, as is thought to be the case, in most women the question arises as to why some women develop implants and others do not. There is increasing largely circumstantial evidence that immunological malfunction may be involved in this selectivity and there may also be a genetic factor.

The pathology of endometriosis is, in essence, simple. The only diagnostic criterion is the presence of histologically recognisable endometrial glands and stroma in an ectopic site (Figure 7.33). Unfortunately, however, the situation is complicated by the tendency towards haemorrhage that is such a characteristic feature of endometriosis. Bleeding into the lesion itself can cause considerable damage and a 'self-destruction' of the endometrial tissue, thus destroying the specific histological findings. Futhermore, haemorrhage into the surrounding tissues releases free iron which is intensely fibrogenic and promotes dense adhesions that tend to obscure the primary lesion.

The early stages of ovarian endometriosis appear to the naked eye as reddish-blue surface implants, which may be raised or dimpled and can measure from 1mm to 5mm across. It is usual for tiny cysts to appear and these progressively enlarge and grow into ovarian tissue, usually reaching a size of 2–5cm across but occasionally attaining a diameter of up to 10cm. The cysts have a smooth or granular lining which is brownish-yellow and their walls, originally thin, become eventually

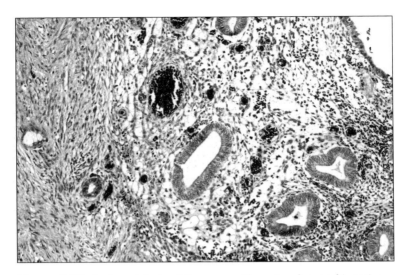

Figure 7.33 Endometriosis of the ovary. There is a focus of inactive endometrial tissue on the ovarian surface.

thick and fibrotic. Their content of old, semi-fluid or inspissated, blood commonly has a dark brown or black appearance, a feature which has led to the use of the terms 'chocolate' or 'tarry' cyst. There is a marked tendency for blood to leak out from endometriotic cysts and this results in the formation of firm adhesions which bind the enlarged ovary down to the posterior surface of either the broad ligament or the uterus. Any attempt at separating the ovary from these structures leads to an escape of brown or black cyst contents. Peritubal adhesions are frequently seen and the tubes may be kinked and distorted. However, the tubal ostia are usually patent and the tubal lumen is rarely obstructed.

The histological diagnosis of ovarian endometriosis is readily made if endometrial glands and stroma are still present in recognisable form in the lesion. It is, however, by no means unusual for the endometrial lining of the cysts either to be so attenuated as to be unrecognisable as such, or to be largely or completely lost (Figure 7.34). If the endometrial lining has been totally destroyed, the appearance will be that of a simple haemorrhagic cyst lined by granulation tissue and with a fibrous wall in which aggregates of iron-containing macrophages are usually present. Under these circumstances it is justifiable to conclude that the appearances are 'compatible with a diagnosis of endometriosis' or even to make a diagnosis of 'presumptive endometriosis'. Any endometrial

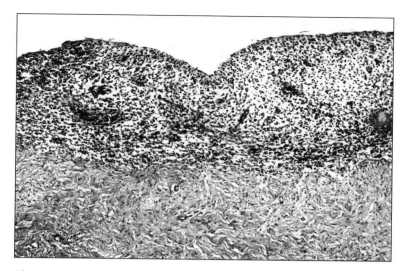

Figure 7.34 The wall of an endometriotic cyst of the ovary. The cyst is lined by non-specific granulation tissue and endometrial stroma: the wall, below, is formed of fibrous tissue.

tissue that is present may show the full range of normal cyclical changes but can appear either to be inactive or to show only proliferative activity. Under the latter circumstances there may be a progression to a simple or atypical hyperplasia.

Extraovarian pelvic endometriosis, for example in the uterosacral and round ligaments, pouch of Douglas, rectovaginal septum or on the surface of the uterus, is seen as multiple bluish-red nodules, patches, or cysts, almost invariably with accompanying fibrous adhesions. The lesions are usually small but ligamentous foci may attain a size sufficient to be easily palpable and endometriotic foci in the rectovaginal septum cannot only lead to fixation of the rectum but can extend into the vaginal vault or the rectum to form small haemorrhagic nodules or polyps.

Occasionally, an *in situ* adenocarcinoma is encountered in an endometriotic focus. Overt malignant change gives rise to an endometrioid adenocarcinoma, which is usually of the conventional variety, though any of the many morphological variants of this type of neoplasm, particularly clear-cell adenocarcinomas, can also arise in endometriotic foci. Extra-ovarian endometriosis can also, uncommonly, undergo neoplastic change and give rise to an endometrioid or clear-cell adenocarcinoma in such sites as the uterine ligaments, pouch of Douglas, rectovaginal septum or bladder.

8 Abnormalities related to pregnancy

Ectopic pregnancy

In approximately one percent of all recognised pregnancies the conceptus implants in a site other than the uterine cavity. The vast majority (95–97%) of such ectopic gestations occur in the fallopian tube. Less common sites are the ovary, cervix and peritoneal cavity and occasional cases of implantation occur in the vagina, liver or spleen.

Tubal pregnancies are predisposed to by any factor which impairs the ability of the tube to transport the fertilised ovum. Hence congenital abnormalities of the tube, failed tubal sterilisation, the use of a progesterone-only contraceptive pill, salpingitis isthmica nodosa, reconstructive tubal surgery and, most importantly, post-inflammatory tubal damage are all associated with an increased incidence of tubal pregnancy. In about 50% of such pregnancies the tube is, however, fully normal.

It has been argued that in such cases conception occurred during a cycle in which there was delayed ovulation and a short, inadequate luteal phase. Consequently, when the fertilised ovum reached the uterine cavity it had not yet developed to a stage when it was secreting enough hCG to prevent decay of the corpus luteum and was flushed back into the tube by a reflux of menstrual blood subsequent to menstrual bleeding. This hypothesis is supported by the fact that tubal gestation occurs only in species which menstruate and by the not uncommon finding of the corpus luteum of pregnancy on the opposite side to that of a tube containing a pregnancy. This latter phenomenon could, however, also be due to transuterine or transperitoneal migration of the fertilised ovum into the contralateral tube where, because of its relatively advanced stage of development, it implants.

If pregnancy occurs in a woman using an IUCD there is a higher than usual risk that it will be ectopically situated. This is not because such a device causes an ectopic pregnancy, it simply fails to prevent extrauterine implantation as effectively as it inhibits implantation within the uterus.

Within the tube, the fertilised ovum implants most commonly in the ampulla. Implantation occurs in exactly the same manner in the tube as it does in the uterus but, nevertheless, a high proportion of tubal pregnancies abort at an early stage. This may be because the conceptus has implanted on the plicae, which offer an inadequate site for placentation or because trophoblastic invasion of the tubal vessels leads to intramural and intraluminal haemorrhage. Following early abortion the products of conception may be retained in the tube as a form of 'chronic ectopic', be expelled via the uterus or gradually absorbed.

Tubal rupture complicates about 50% of tubal pregnancies and appears to be due partly to the limited distensibility of the tube and partly to transmural spread of invading extravillous trophoblast with serosal penetration. Rupture is usually acute and is accompanied by intraperitoneal bleeding and the clinical features of an acute abdomen. Less commonly, there is a slow leakage of tubal contents and blood from the tube, which results in a gradually enlarging peritubal haematoma and causes dense adhesions between the tube and surrounding structures such as omentum and intestines. Occasionally the ureters are obstructed by involvement in this peritubal mass.

Tubal rupture is usually accompanied by fetal death but occasionally the fetus retains sufficient attachment to its blood supply to maintain its viability with the trophoblast growing out through the rupture site and forming a secondary placental site in the abdomen or broad ligament. A secondary abdominal pregnancy of this type may proceed virtually to term.

Trophoblastic disease

The term 'trophoblastic disease' is, by convention, restricted to hydatidiform moles, choriocarcinoma and the placental site trophoblastic tumour.

HYDATIDIFORM MOLE

Only within recent years has it been recognised that there are two fundamentally different types of mole, the complete and partial forms.

Complete hydatidiform mole

Complete moles complicate about one in 1500 gestations in most western countries but are encountered, for currently unknown reasons, much more frequently in many parts of Africa, Asia and Latin America. They occur particularly in the two extremes of the reproductive era, in women aged less than 18 or more than 40 years, and usually present either as an abortion or as first-trimester vaginal

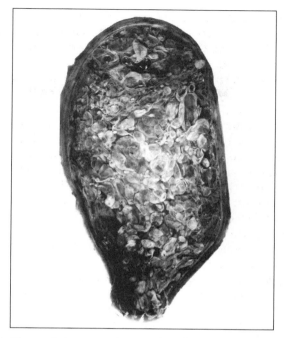

Figure 8.1 A complete hydatidiform mole which fills, and distends, the uterine cavity.

bleeding. A complete hydatidiform mole (Figure 8.1) forms a bulky mass, sometimes weighing as much as 2000g, which, when *in situ*, fills and distends the uterine cavity. No fetus is present and no normal placental tissue is seen, but all the chorionic villi are swollen and distended to give a 'bunch of grapes' appearance. Histologically (Figure 8.2), the villi are devoid of fetal vessels and are markedly oedematous, many showing central liquefaction. A constant feature is atypical growth of the villous trophoblast. Some pleomorphism is often apparent in the proliferating trophoblast but it is the pattern, rather than the degree, of proliferation of trophoblastic cells which is atypical, this being either circumferential or multifocal in nature rather than polar, as in the normal first-trimester placenta.

Cytogenetic studies have shown that 85% of complete hydatidiform moles have a 46XX chromosomal constitution, both X chromosomes being of paternal (androgenetic) origin. It is thought that this is the result of penetration of a 'dead' ovum, which then duplicates without cytokinesis. Fifteen per cent of complete moles have, however, a 46XY chromosomal constitution, both chromosomes again being derived

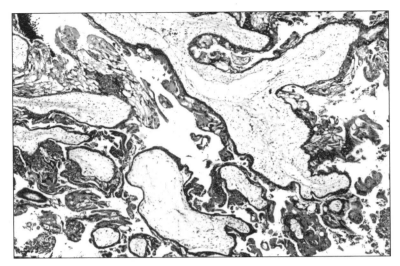

Figure 8.2 A complete hydatidiform mole. All the villi are abnormal and some show central cisternal change: there is an abnormal pattern of trophoblastic proliferation.

from the father. It is believed that this type of complete mole results from the entry of two haploid sperms, one X and the other Y, into an abnormal ovum with subsequent fusion and replication. All XY moles are therefore dispermic (or 'heterologous') and it is now clear that although the vast majority of 46XX moles are monospermic (homozygous), a small proportion resemble the XY moles in being dispermic, presumably because of the entry of two, rather than one, haploid X sperms into a defective ovum.

Hydatidiform moles are a particular form of pregnancy which ends in abortion rather than, as is often implied, a benign neoplasm. Nevertheless, women who have had a complete mole have a much greater risk of subsequently developing a choriocarcinoma (in the region of two to three percent) than do women who have had a normal pregnancy. Attempts have been made to identify those moles most likely to be followed by a choriocarcinoma by grading the degree of trophoblastic hyperplasia. It is maintained that the more marked the degree of trophoblastic proliferation the greater the risk of eventual choriocarcinoma. Attempts to apply this principle in practice have, however, failed to confirm that the histological features of a complete mole are of any prognostic value and, indeed, reliance upon morphological criteria is potentially dangerous, leading to a false sense of security in some cases and to overtreatment in others. It is now agreed that all women should, after evacuation of a mole, be followed up with serial estimations of hCG levels, surveillance being maintained until, and for up to one year after, levels of this placental hormone have returned to normal.

Women in whom hCG values remain elevated or increase during follow-up are classed as having 'persistent trophoblastic disease'. This condition may be due to the persistence of residual molar villi or proliferating trophoblast, the development of an invasive mole (see below), or the development of a choriocarcinoma. In most cases no attempt is made to establish a specific diagnosis and the patients are treated, empirically but successfully, with a short course of chemotherapy.

Partial hydatidiform mole

In a partial mole, vesicular change affects only a proportion of the villous population of a placenta. The macroscopic appearances are therefore those of a largely normal placenta in which, however, a variable number of distended villi are often, though not invariably, present. Histologically (Figure 8.3), only a proportion of the villi are distended by oedema fluid, these being intermingled with fully normal villi. The scattered vesicular villi have a markedly irregular outline and show atypical trophoblastic proliferation, usually multifocal in nature and commonly less marked than that seen in a complete mole.

The vast majority of partial hydatidiform moles are associated with a

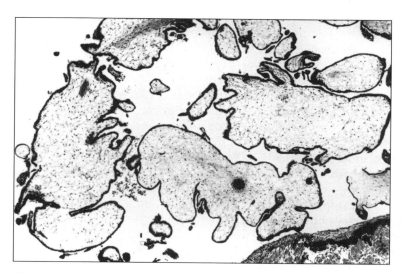

Figure 8.3 A partial hydatidiform mole. The villi vary in size, some being normal and others large with irregular outlines.

fetal triploidy, a small minority having a tetraploid, trisomic, or diploid chromosomal constitution. Not all triploid conceptions result in moles and it is now known that if the additional chromosomes are of maternal origin a normal placenta will result, whereas if the excess chromosomal load is paternally derived a partial mole will develop.

The natural history of a partial mole and the magnitude of the risk of subsequent choriocarcinoma have not yet been adequately defined, but it is now clear that a partial mole can be invasive and followed by persistent trophoblastic disease. Hence women who have had a partial mole should be followed up in exactly the same way as those with complete moles.

Invasive hydatidiform mole

In five to ten percent of moles, either complete or partial, molar villi invade the myometrium, sometimes even penetrating the uterine wall to extend into the broad ligament. Myometrial vessels may also be breached by the invasive villous tissue. A deeply invasive mole usually becomes clinically apparent several weeks after apparently complete evacuation of a mole from the uterus, the patient commonly presenting with haemorrhage. Hysterectomy at this stage will reveal intramyometrial haemorrhagic foci and, on microscopy, vesicular villi are seen in the uterine wall and within myometrial vessels. The villous tissue within the vessels can be transported as emboli to sites such as the lung or vagina where they may continue to grow. Any pulmonary nodules are usually only apparent radiologically but vaginal lesions present as haemorrhagic submucosal nodules. Biopsy of these extrauterine lesions will show molar villi, a finding which excludes a diagnosis of choriocarcinoma.

An invasive mole is not a malignant lesion. Normal placental villi can penetrate deeply into the myometrium, as in the condition of placenta increta, and trophoblastic transportation to extrauterine sites occurs in every pregnancy. An invasive mole simply represents, therefore, a molar version of placenta increta with associated trophoblastic deportation.

In practice, the diagnosis of an invasive mole is now largely obsolete, for patients with this type of mole are usually diagnosed as having persistent trophoblastic disease prior to development of symptoms and are treated by chemotherapy.

CHORIOCARCINOMA

This is a malignant neoplasm of trophoblast and has a unique status because, being of fetal origin, it is the only human tumour which is, in effect, an allograft. Choriocarcinoma is extremely rare in western countries, complicating approximately one in 45,000 pregnancies, although, as with the hydatidiform mole, it is much more common in many parts of Africa, Asia and South America. Approximately 50% of choriocarcinomas follow a hydatidiform mole, 30% develop after an abortion and 20% occur after a normal pregnancy. The time-interval between the antecedent pregnancy and the development of a chorio-carcinoma is very variable, ranging from a few months to 15 years.

A choriocarcinoma forms single or multiple haemorrhagic nodules within the uterus. These are well delineated and consist of a central area of haemorrhagic necrosis and a peripheral rim of viable tumour tissue. The central necrosis is due to the fact that a choriocarcinoma has no intrinsic blood supply, relying for its oxygenation and nutrition on its ability to invade and permeate the maternal vasculature. Histologically (Figure 8.4), the tumour has a pattern which recapitu-lates that of the early implanting blastocyst, central cores of cyto-trophoblastic cells being surrounded by a peripheral rim of syncytiotrophoblast. The trophoblastic cells do not differ significantly from those of a normal blastocyst and mitotic activity is rarely exten-sive. Villi are not present in a choriocarcinoma and, indeed, the pres-ence of villous structures refutes this diagnosis.

The capacity of malignant trophoblast to invade vessels offers an adequate explanation for the primarily vascular dissemination of this tumour, spread occurring at an early stage to the brain, lungs, liver,

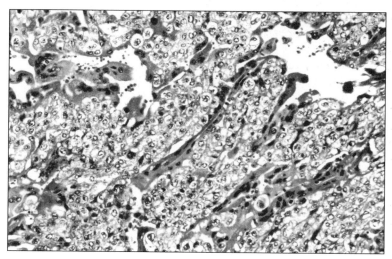

Figure 8.4 Choriocarcinoma. The neoplasm is composed of two types of cell, the darkly-staining syncytiotrophoblast and the pale-staining cytotrophoblast.

kidneys and gastrointestinal tract. It is therefore not surprising that choriocarcinoma was, in the past, a highly lethal neoplasm with a mortality little short of 100% and with death occurring in months rather than in years. For no other neoplasm, however, has the advent of chemotherapy more radically altered the prognosis, with over 85% of patients now being permanently cured with cytotoxic drugs.

PLACENTAL SITE TROPHOBLASTIC TUMOUR

This neoplasm originates from the extravillous trophoblastic cells which are normally present in the decidua and myometrium of the placental bed, and form the placental site reaction. A placental site trophoblastic tumour usually occurs after a normal gestation and symptoms such as abnormal bleeding or amenorrhoea become apparent months or years after the pregnancy.

The tumour forms a nodular tan or yellow mass which shows little necrosis or haemorrhage. Histologically (Figure 8.5), trophoblastic cells, predominantly of the mononuclear cytotrophoblastic type, infiltrate between myometrial fibres in sheets, cords and islands. Some multinucleated cells are usually present but the bilaminar pattern of a choriocarcinoma is not seen. Vascular permeation by tumour cells is seen but the massive intravascular growth typical of a choriocarcinoma is not apparent.

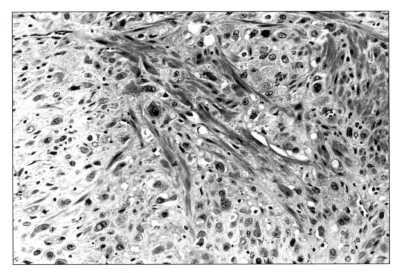

Figure 8.5 Placental site trophoblastic tumour. The myometrium is infiltrated by cords and sheets of extravillous cytotrophoblastic cells: there is no necrosis or haemorrhage.

Most of these tumours are cured by simple hysterectomy, but about ten percent extend beyond the uterus and behave in a malignant fashion. In general, neoplasms with an abundance of mitotic figures are most likely to pursue a malignant course but there is no histological feature that can predict malignant behaviour with certainty. Treatment of malignant cases is currently unsatisfactory, for these neoplasms do not respond well to the therapeutic regime that has met with such success in the treatment of choriocarcinoma.

Pathology of the placenta

DEVELOPMENTAL ABNORMALITIES

The only common developmental abnormality of the placenta is extra-chorial placentation, in which the chorionic plate, from which the villi arise, is smaller than the basal plate, the transition from villous to non-villous chorion taking place not at the placental margin but at some distance inside the circumference of the fetal surface of the placenta (Figure 8.6). If this transition is marked by a flat ring of membranes, the placenta is classed as 'circummarginate', whereas if this ring has a raised, rolled edge, the placenta is 'circumvallate'. The circummarginate form is devoid of any functional importance and, although circumvallate placentation is associated more frequently than can be explained by chance alone with a rather small baby and, possibly, with a slight excess of congenital malformations, it is not associated with any excess of perinatal mortality. Other aberrant forms of placentation are either relatively common but functionally unimportant, for example the bilobate placenta and accessory lobe, or functionally important but excessively rare, such as placenta membranacea and girdle placenta.

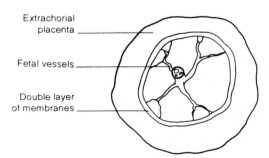

Extrachorial placenta

Fetal vessels

Double layer of membranes

Figure 8.6 Diagrammatic representation of a placenta extrachorialis as viewed from the fetal aspect.

GROSS LESIONS OF THE PLACENTA

A fresh placental infarct is firm and dark red. As it ages, it becomes progressively harder and its colour changes successively to brown, yellow then white, so that an old infarct appears as an amorphous, hard, white plaque (Figure 8.7). Histologically, an early infarct is characterised by aggregation of the villi and early necrotic changes in the villous syncytiotrophoblast. With the passage of time, the infarcted villi undergo a progressive necrobiosis, so that the old infarct consists only of crowded ghost villi.

Small placental infarcts are common and of no importance, but extensive infarction, that is necrosis of more than ten percent of the placenta, is accompanied by a high incidence of fetal hypoxia, growth retardation and intrauterine death. These ill-effects have been thought to be a direct consequence of the loss of viable villous tissue by those who consider that the placenta has little or no functional reserve capacity. However, another common lesion that reduces the number of functioning villi is perivillous fibrin deposition that is sufficiently extensive to appear as either a hard white plaque or an area of irregular whitish mottling. Histologically, such lesions consist of widely separated villi that are entrapped in fibrin, which is filling in and obliterating the intervillous space. The entrapped villi undergo a secondary sclerosis but are not infarcted. Nevertheless, they are excluded from playing any role in maternal–fetal transfer and are just as much lost, in a physiological sense, to the fetus as they would be if they were infarcted. Although perivillous fibrin deposition depletes the population of functional villi, this lesion is of no clinical importance, even when it is extensive enough to functionally inactivate 30% of the villi by entrapment in fibrin.

The ability of the placenta to withstand the loss of one-third of its functioning tissue without any discernible effect on fetal growth or development shows that the placenta quite obviously has a consider-

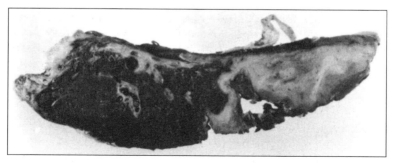

Figure 8.7 An old placental infarct: this is seen as a whitish plaque.

able functional reserve capacity, but it still leaves unexplained why loss of villi due to infarction poses a grave threat to the fetus while a similar, or even greater, loss of villi due to entrapment in fibrin is of no consequence. This paradox is more apparent than real if the pathogenesis of these two lesions is considered. Perivillous fibrin deposition is due to haemodynamic turbulence within the intervillous space, with eddy stasis of maternal blood and laying down of fibrin; therefore, the greater the quantity of maternal blood entering the closed, irregular intervillous space per unit of time, the greater the risk of turbulence and hence of perivillous fibrin deposition. This lesion tends to occur, therefore, in placentas with a particularly good maternal uteroplacental blood flow. Infarction, however, is usually due to thrombosis of a maternal uteroplacental vessel, and therefore extensive infarction implies widespread thrombosis within the maternal vasculature. This would not be expected to occur in a healthy maternal tree, and it is therefore no coincidence that extensive infarction is virtually confined to placentas from women with pre-eclampsia, a condition in which an acute 'atherosis' is found in the uteroplacental vessels and which predisposes to thrombosis. Far more importantly, however, in pre-eclamptic women, whether thrombosis occurs or not, there is a severely-restricted maternal blood flow to the placenta (the reasons for which are discussed later) and it is this limitation of maternal blood flow that is the real cause of the apparent complications of placental infarction.

The true significance of extensive placental infarction is therefore that it is the visible hallmark of a markedly abnormal maternal vasculature and of a severely-restricted maternal-uteroplacental blood flow. It is true that under these circumstances the placental infarction may further worsen the situation, but the infarction *per se* is not the primary cause of the fetal complications and would be of little or no importance if it occurred in a placenta with an adequate maternal blood supply.

Most other macroscopic lesions of the placenta are of no functional significance and can be ignored. Large retroplacental haematomas, widespread thrombosis of fetal vessels, maternal floor infarction and large haemangiomas can be of clinical importance but these are rare. Otherwise the various plaques, thrombi and cysts that can occur in the placenta lack clinical importance as does gross placental calcification.

EXTRAVILLOUS TROPHOBLAST AND THE PATHOLOGY OF THE UTEROPLACENTAL VESSELS

It is difficult to accept that most cases of 'placental insufficiency' are caused by intrinsic placental damage and it is becoming increasingly clear that the common factor in most cases of presumed placental inadequacy is a reduced maternal blood flow to the fetoplacental unit. The placenta establishes its own blood supply as a result of invasion of the spiral arteries in the placental bed by extravillous trophoblast which destroys the muscle and elastic tissue of the media of these vessels and replaces these components with fibrinoid material. This process results in the conversion of the thick-walled, muscular spiral arteries into thin-walled, flaccid, sac-like uteroplacental vessels which can passively dilate to accommodate the great increase in maternal blood flow to the placenta which is required as pregnancy progresses. This physiological change within the spiral arteries occurs in two stages. During the first 12 weeks of gestation the extravillous trophoblast invades only the intradecidual portion of the spiral arteries of the placental bed but, after a resting phase, the extravillous trophoblast invades the intra-myometrial segments of these vessels between the 14th and 16th weeks of pregnancy.

The factors controlling and limiting intravascular invasion by extravillous trophoblast are unknown, but the crucial importance of this process is shown by the finding that in women destined to develop pre-eclampsia in the later stages of pregnancy, and in many cases of normotensive intrauterine fetal growth retardation, there is a partial failure of placentation, which results in a markedly restricted blood flow to the placenta. This failure has two components. First, while in a normal pregnancy all the spiral arteries in the placental bed are invaded by trophoblast, this process occurs in only a proportion of these vessels in such patients, with a significant fraction of the placental bed arteries showing a complete absence of physiological change. Second, in those arteries that are invaded by extravillous trophoblast, the first stage in this process occurs normally with trophoblast evoking physiological changes in their intradecidual segments. There is subsequently a complete failure of the second stage, with endovascular trophoblast failing to advance into the intramyometrial portion of these vessels. Hence, in these women there is an incomplete transformation of the spiral arteries to uteroplacental vessels, an abnormality which has been clearly shown to result in a restriction of the maternal blood flow to the placenta and which will restrict the ability of the mother to provide the fetus with an adequate supply of oxygen and nutrients. A reduced uteroplacental blood flow is, in itself, an adequate cause for all the placental abnormalities seen in pre-eclampsia and for intrauterine growth retardation. The decreased maternal blood flow also serves as the basis for the maternal syndrome of pre-eclampsia in so far as a factor appears to be released from the ischaemic placenta which causes widespread maternal endothelial damage.

Most cases of apparent placental insufficiency are, therefore, in reality examples of maternal vascular insufficiency.

PLACENTAL INFECTION

Infective agents may reach the placenta either from the maternal bloodstream to produce a villitis or may ascend from the birth canal to produce a chorioamnionitis.

Villitis may be due to placental involvement in specific maternal infections, such as rubella virus, toxoplasmosis, listeriosis, syphilis, or cytomegalovirus, but such conditions account for only a small proportion of cases of villitis, the vast majority of which are of unknown cause. There is a clear association between the presence of a villitis and a high incidence of fetal intrauterine growth retardation, although the nature of this relationship is obscure. Most cases of villitis are focal with only a small proportion of the villi showing any evidence of either a healed or an active inflammatory process. This degree of villous damage is unlikely to impair the functional reserve capacity of the placenta and it is possible that the low birth weight in such cases is due not to villous damage but to infection crossing the placenta and affecting the fetus by inhibiting DNA synthesis. Villitis may thus simply serve as an indicator of possible fetal infection.

A chorioamnionitis, characterised by polymorphonuclear leucocytic infiltration of the extraplacental and placental membranes, is due to an ascending infection which is commonly of polymicrobial aetiology. Prolonged membrane rupture predisposes to chorioamnionitis but chorioamnionitis can also occur in the presence of intact membranes.

Ascending infections can cause both premature onset of labour and premature rupture of the membranes and chorioamnionitis is a major aetiological factor in preterm labour, particularly before the 35th week of gestation. The mechanism by which an ascending infection stimulates the premature onset of labour is still uncertain, but it is thought that cytokines produced by activated macrophages stimulate excess synthesis of prostaglandins, which are of vital importance in initiating parturition, by amniotic and decidual cells. Some cases of preterm delivery associated with an ascending infection are, however, due not to premature onset of labour but to premature rupture of the membranes which may be the result of the combination of release of elastases and collagenases from the neutrophil polymorphonuclear leucocytes infiltrating the membranes and the secretion of proteolytic enzymes by bacteria.

NON-TROPHOBLASTIC TUMOURS OF THE PLACENTA

The only common non-trophoblastic tumour of the placenta is the haemangioma or 'chorioangioma'. Haemangiomas, usually single but occasionally multiple, are present in one percent of placentas. The vast majority are small and intraplacental where they form well-demar-

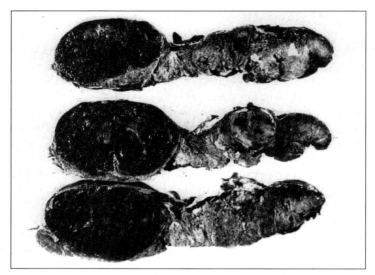

Figure 8.8 A large intra-placental haemangioma (to the left).

cated, rounded, usually red, intraparenchymal nodules. The uncommon large haemangiomas (Figure 8.8), measuring more than 5cm in diameter, are usually seen as protruberances on the fetal surface of the placenta. Occasionally they can be found on the maternal surface, where they often appear to replace an entire lobe, or in the membranes attached to the main placental mass only by a vascular pedicle. Histologically, placental haemangiomas have a microscopic appearance identical to that seen in similar tumours elsewhere in the body.

The vast majority of placental haemangiomas are of no clinical importance, but a very small minority – those measuring more than 5cm in diameter – may be associated with a variety of complications that can affect the mother, fetus, or neonate. There is a high incidence of polyhydramnios in association with large haemangiomas. The cause of this is obscure but it may precipitate premature labour. Large tumours are also associated, as are multiple small tumours within a single placenta, with an increased incidence of intrauterine fetal hypoxia, intrauterine growth retardation and intrauterine death. All these complications have been attributed to the fact that a considerable proportion of the fetal blood passes through the tumour, rather than through functional placental tissue, and is therefore returned to the fetus in an unoxygenated and nutrient-poor state. The neonate whose placenta contains a large haemangioma is also subject to a number of complications, usually of a transitory nature, which are a direct consequence of the placental tumour. Prominent among these is cardiomegaly; this is probably a result of the increased fetal cardiac output required for pumping blood through the haemangioma, which in haemodynamic terms can be considered a peripheral arteriovenous shunt. Neonatal oedema is sometimes a manifestation of cardiac failure but can also be due to hypoalbuminaemia which results either from transudation of protein from the surface vessels of the tumour or from chronic fetal–maternal bleeding from the haemangioma. Neonatal anaemia can be a result of sequestration of fetal erythrocytes with the tumour, a massive feto-maternal bleed from the haemangioma or a microangiopathic haemolytic anaemia induced by injury inflicted on fetal red blood cells as they transverse the labyrinthine vascular channels of the tumour. Neonatal thrombocytopenia can also be due to platelet injury within the tumour vessels but is sometimes a manifestation of disseminated intravascular coagulation triggered by a thromboplastic substance released from the haemangioma.

THE PLACENTA IN TWIN PREGNANCY (Figure 8.9)

Dizygotic twins may have two separate and discrete placentas, each with its own amniotic sac (dichorionic-diamniotic pregnancy). The two placentas may, however, apparently fuse, though there will still be two

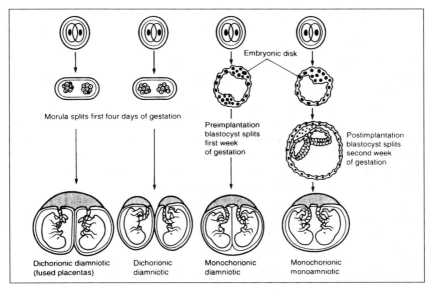

Figure 8.9 Diagrammatic representation of the development and placentation of monozygotic twins.

amniotic sacs. Monozygotic twins may also have separate placentas and amniotic sacs but in some cases there is a single placenta with two amniotic sacs (monochorionic-diamniotic pregnancy) whilst in others there is a single placenta and a single amniotic sac (monochorionic-monoamniotic pregnancy). A distinction between fused dichorionic-diamniotic and monochorionic-diamniotic placentas can be made by examining the septum between the two amniotic sacs (or the T zone at the base of this septum). Chorionic tissue is present between the two layers of the septum in a dichorionic-diamniotic placentation but is absent from the septum of a monochorionic-diamniotic twin placenta (Figure 8.10).

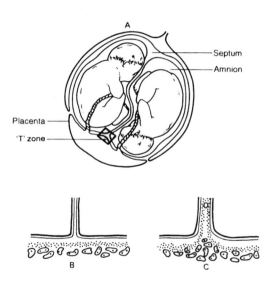

Figure 8.10

(A) Diagrammatic representation of the base of the septum in a diamniotic twin placenta. (B) Diagrammatic representation of the base of the septum in a monochorionic-diamniotic twin placenta: the septum consists only of two layers of amnion. (C) Diagrammatic representation of the base of the septum in a dichorionic-diamniotic twin placenta: chorionic tissue is present in the septum between the two layers of the amnion.

Vascular anastomoses between the twin circulations are often present in diamniotic-monochorionic placentas and these can lead to the twin-to-twin transfusion syndrome in which the recipient twin develops polyhydramnios and cardiomegaly as a result of vascular overload whilst the donor twin develops anaemia and oligohydramnios. A transfusion syndrome can lead to the death of the donor twin and such fetal demise can be complicated by brain damage in the surviving twin because of hypovolaemic shock resulting from blood draining into the dead twin's resistance-free vascular bed.

Twin-to-twin transfusion rarely occurs in monochorionic-monoamniotic placentas but entanglement of the cords leads to a high fetal mortality in this form of twin placentation.

9 Cervical cytology

The cervical smear (Papanicolaou [Pap] test) is a simple, safe and inexpensive method of detecting cervical pre-malignancy. Providing the smear is correctly taken and is interpreted with skill and care, it will provide the gynaecologist with reliable information about the state of the cervix and enable him to reassure his patient about her risk of cervical neoplasia with a high degree of confidence.

In this section, key aspects of cervical cytology are described, including: indications for taking a cervical smear, instructions for specimen collection, the interpretation of the results of the cervical smear test and the factors which influence the accuracy of the test. Reference is made to the management of women within the national cervical screening programme where this is relevant to clinical practice.

Indications for a cervical smear test

There are three reasons for taking a cervical smear:
1 Population screening for cervical pre-cancer and early cervical cancer.
2 As a limited part of the investigation of a woman suspected on clinical grounds of having cervical cancer.
3 As part of the follow-up of patients following treatment of CIN.

POPULATION SCREENING

The cervical smear test is offered world-wide, but unfortunately rarely in underdeveloped countries, as a method of screening healthy women for preinvasive and early invasive cancer of the cervix. In most countries, cervical screening is opportunistic and a cervical smear test is only available on request. In many developed countries, however, screening is highly organised and well women are invited at regular intervals to attend a screening clinic for their smear test. The intervals between smears affect the protective value of the test (Table 9.1). From the table it can be seen that the shorter the interval between smears, the greater the protection afforded to the woman.

Table 9.1 Incidence of invasive squamous cell carcinoma of the cervix uteri following two or more normal smears, as a proportion of the incidence in a comparable unscreened population

Time since last smear (months)	Proportional incidence
0–11	0.06
12–23	0.08
24–35	0.12
36–47	0.19
48–59	0.26
60–71	0.28
72–119	0.63
120+	-1.00

Table 9.2 The effectiveness of different screening policies. Proportionate reduction in incidence of invasive squamous cell carcinoma of the cervix uteri assuming 100% compliance, based on Tables 9.1 and 9.3

Policy	Age group	% reduction in cumulative rate in age group	Numbers of smears per woman
Every 10 years	25–64	64	5
Every 5 years	35–64	70	6
Every 5 years	25–64	82	8
Every 5 years	20–64	84	9
Every 3 years	35–64	78	10
Every 3 years	25–64	90	13
Every 3 years	20–64	91	15
Every year	20–64	93	45

In countries such as the UK, Denmark and the Netherlands with organised screening programmes the interval between tests is three or five years. The frequency of screening in these countries is largely determined by the resources available for the screening programme. Where resources are limited, it has been found that screening every fifth year with a compliance rate of 80% is a much more effective way of reducing cancer mortality and morbidity than annual or three-yearly screening of a small proportion of women at risk.

The target population can only be defined in terms of age. Attempts to define 'at risk' groups using other parameters, such as smoking habits or sexual activity, are theoretically appealing but impossible to implement in clinical practice. In most centres in the UK, a cervical smear test is offered every three years to all women aged between 20 and 35, and every five years for women aged between 35 and 64. Cervical cytology ceases in women with a normal smear history at the age of 65. Thus women who are participating in the programme can expect to have 12 smears in a lifetime and have an 84% reduced risk of developing cervical cancer (Table 9.2).

In some cytology screening centres, a second smear is taken one year after the first negative smear. This has not been shown to be effective and should be discouraged. Moreover, some clinicians tend to take an additional smear when a women is starting oral contraceptive therapy or having an IUCD inserted even though the woman may have had a negative smear within three years and is asymptomatic. Similarly, an additional smear is sometimes taken opportunistically when a woman is pregnant, has genital warts or herpes, or admits to being a heavy smoker. In none of these instances is the additional smear justified providing the women is asymptomatic, is participating in the routine screening programme and has had a negative smear within the previous three (or five) years.

DIAGNOSTIC TEST

A cervical smear test is a useful adjunct to inspection of the cervix in women who have symptoms or signs suggestive of cervical cancer, such as postcoital or postmenopausal bleeding. It can confirm a clinical suspicion of cancer. However, it must be remembered that *colposcopy* and *biopsy* are indicated in cases where there is a clinical suspicion of cancer, *even if the smear report is negative.* A cervical smear can be misleading in patients with advanced cancer as smears from such cases may contain blood, inflammatory cells and necrotic debris only.

FOLLOW-UP AFTER TREATMENT OF CIN

Cervical smears are mandatory in monitoring patients who have received treatment for CIN. By means of cervical cytology it is possible to detect evidence of residual disease due to incomplete clearance following ablative or excisional treatment and also to detect signs of recurrence. The protocol used varies but an acceptable regime is as follows: taking a smear four to six months after initial colposcopy and ablation or excision therapy, repeat at 12 months after the initial treatment and thereafter annually. After five negative smears the interval between smears can be extended to that applied to patients in the general population. Although protocols such as this are widely followed, recent published work has shown recurrences of CIN or the development of invasive disease up to ten years after initial treatment and although no national guidelines have yet been issued with regard to any changes in follow-up protocols there is a possibility that in the future follow-up will need to be extended to up to ten years.

In some centres, a cervical smear is taken routinely at colposcopy, even though the patient presents at the colposcopy clinic because she has an abnormal smear. The argument for doing this is twofold: firstly, the smear taken at the time of colposcopy would be taken under optimal conditions and may indicate the presence of a more advanced squamous or glandular lesion than the original smear; and secondly, the results of the cervical smear tests are especially useful if colposcopic examination and biopsy fail to reveal a significant lesion. An alternative viewpoint is put by some gynaecological pathologists who prefer biopsy specimens from the cervices not subjected to the superficial trauma of smear-taking, as such trauma can remove the surface layers of epithelium and render the biopsies more difficult to interpret. If a smear has been taken within six months and was deemed as 'adequate' it is commonly advised that the smear does not need to be repeated at the time of colposcopy. In deciding which of these two approaches to adopt it is, of course, essential that advice be sought from the gynaecological pathologist and cytopathologists providing the service and their advice be adhered to.

Specimen collection

The cervical smear test is based on the knowledge that tumour cells lose the cohesive properties of normal cells and are therefore readily dislodged when the cervix is scraped. In practice, the earliest and smallest neoplastic lesion can be detected by examination of the smear before it is visible to the naked eye. Thus, cytological investigation can provide a very sensitive method of detecting neoplasia.

Several methods have been described for obtaining cytological samples from the uterine cervix. These include cervical scrape and endocervical brush techniques.

THE CERVICAL SCRAPE

Numerous studies have shown that this is the most efficient single method of detecting malignant and clinically unsuspected invasive cancer of the cervix. An excellent illustrated account of the technique

Figure 9.1
Equipment needed
for taking a
cervical smear.

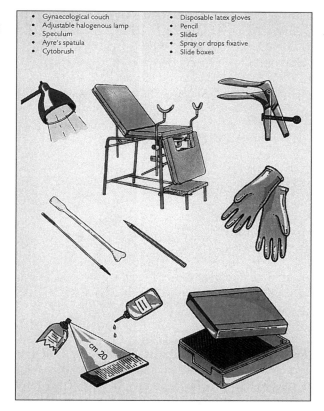

- Gynaecological couch
- Adjustable halogenous lamp
- Speculum
- Ayre's spatula
- Cytobrush

- Disposable latex gloves
- Pencil
- Slides
- Spray or drops fixative
- Slide boxes

is available from the British Society for Clinical Cytology[1]. The equipment required includes a speculum, cervical spatula, glass slides with
frosted end, fixative, pencil, request form, latex gloves and box for
transporting the slides (Figure 9.1).

Taking the smear

The cervical scrape is obtained under direct vision with the vaginal
speculum in position and the patient in the left lateral or dorsal position. Good illumination of the cervix is essential and a speculum of
suitable size should be used. The smear should be taken before
bimanual examination of the cervix to prevent bleeding and before the
application of acetic acid if the smear is taken at colposcopy. Lubricant

[1]   *Taking a Cervical Smear*, BSCC Handbook and Video available from the British Society for
      Clinical Cytology, c/o Thorn EMI, Central Research Laboratories, Dawley Road, Hayes,
      Middlesex UB3 1HH, UK.

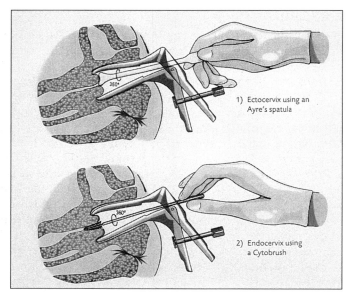

Figure 9.2 Technique for taking a smear (i) cervical scrape, (ii) cervical brush.

apart from water should be avoided or used very sparingly and the cervix must be clearly visualised before the smear is taken. It should not be wiped or cleansed in any way prior to sampling.

The tip of the spatula should be inserted into the cervical os and rotated gently but firmly through 360° as shown in Figure 9.2. The cervical mucus and cellular material on the spatula is spread evenly across the glass slide which has been previously labelled in pencil with the patient's name. The cells on the slide must be fixed by spraying or immersion in 95% ethanol. On no account should smears be allowed to dry before fixation as such 'air drying' impairs the staining properties of the cells. Once fixation is complete the smears should be placed in an appropriate container and transported to the cytology laboratory or sent by post.

Accompanying details about the patient are essential and must include patient's surname, forename, postal address and date of birth. Specimen type (e.g. brush or scrape) must also be indicated on the request form. Information about the clinical appearance of the cervix and relevant symptoms should be included as should previous smear history and date of last smear if this is available. Details of menstrual history and current methods of contraception are also required. This information will facilitate the correct interpretation of the smear.

Choice of spatula

The aim of the cervical scrape is to obtain a representative sample of cells from the transformation zone. A large number of cervical sampling devices has been developed to try to ensure that this occurs and the choice can be quite bewildering. The Ayre's spatula is widely used in clinical practice but the bi-lobed end, which is ideal for sampling the multiparous premenopausal cervix, is too wide to be inserted into the narrow os of a nulliparous or postmenopausal patient. Alternative spatulae have been designed to deal with such cases and several are shown in Figure 9.3. The Aylesbury spatula, which has an extended tip, has proved an effective sampling device in large-scale clinical trials in the United Kingdom. The rounded end of the spatula is useful for taking samples from women with a patulous os. Plastic spatulae have the advantage over wooden spatulae in that less material is retained on the spatula once the smear is made. On the other hand, plastic spatulae are more likely to cause cervical bleeding than wooden spatulae. It is wise to have a choice of spatulae available for use at a screening clinic so that an optimal sample can be obtained every time.

ENDOCERVICAL BRUSH

The endocervical brush has been developed for sampling the endocervical canal. There are clear indications for its use:

1   When the os is stenosed.

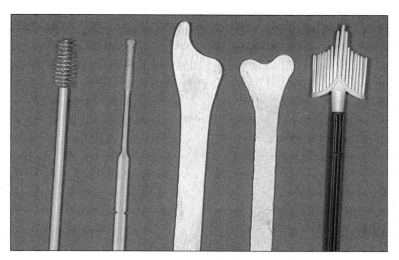

Figure 9.3 Examples of different cervical spatulae and brushes (left to right Medscand cytobrush, CerviBrush, Aylesbury spatula, Ayre's spatula, and spatula /brush combination.

2 When the squamocolumnar junction is high in the endocervical canal, as is usual in the postmenopausal woman.
3 When adenocarcinoma of the cervix is suspected.
4 Following local treatment to the cervix for CIN.

The method of preparing smears from an endocervical brush is shown in Figure 9.2. Immediate fixation in ethanol is essential as air drying distorts the fragile endocervical epithelial cells and makes interpretation difficult. It should be remembered that a cervical brush specimen will not sample the ectocervix, so that the technique on its own is not suitable as a method of screening for cervical cancer. Some gynaecologists prefer to take brush samples routinely together with a cervical scrape to ensure the squamocolumnar junction is sampled. Two smears should then be sent to the laboratory for analysis, each of which should be clearly labelled with regard to the source of cells it contains. A technique has been developed for combining a brush and scrape in a single smear and this is shown in Figure 9.4.

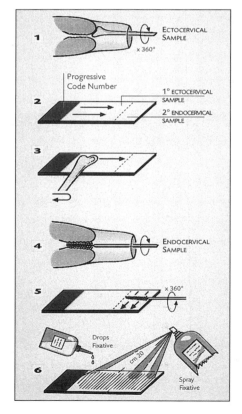

Figure 9.4 Preparation of a cervical smear in which the ectocervical sample and the endocervical brush specimen are combined on one slide.

A survey of different sampling devices was carried out by Buntinx and Brouwers (1996), who compared the yield of histological and cytological abnormalities for a range of devices. Meta-analysis of 30 studies evaluating a range of sampling devices revealed no substantial differences in the yield of mild dysplasia or worse between the Ayres spatula, the Cytobrush, or the cotton swab when used alone. However, the Ayre's spatula, Cytobrush, or cotton swab when used alone performed significantly worse than the combination of any spatula plus the Cytobrush or cotton swab, and this is recommended for screening.

POSTERIOR FORNIX ASPIRATION

This technique was advocated by Papanicolaou in 1943 as a suitable method of obtaining exfoliated cervical cells for the purposes of screening for cervical cancer. It soon became apparent that the cervical scrape provides a better yield of cervical cells than the posterior fornix aspirate and the main use of the latter today is to provide a specimen in the rare cases where the cervix cannot be visualised for anatomical reasons.

VAGINAL VAULT AND LATERAL VAGINAL WALL SMEARS

One of the key uses of cytology is to monitor the progress of patients who have been treated for CIN or invasive cervical cancer by hysterectomy. A smear from the vaginal vault may detect residual cancer or recurrence even though a lesion is not visible to the naked eye. The round end of an Ayre's spatula can be used to obtain the material and smears can be prepared and fixed as for a cervical smear in the usual way.

The preparation and interpretation of cervical smears

It is important for the gynaecologist to be aware of the procedures for processing smears once they arrive at the laboratory. The smears are stained with the Papanicolaou stain which is designed to display epithelial cell morphology and permits visualisation of the nucleus and cytoplasm of the cell. Staining may be carried out on an automated staining machine or manually, but in either event the nuclear chromatin and nuclear membrane should be crisp and clearly defined and the chromatin stained a blue-black colour. The cytoplasm should stain a delicate blue or pink. Nuclear cytoplasmic ratios are clearly important features for the cytologist since alteration of the normal ratios is a signal that the cells may be neoplastic.

The Papanicolaou stain has another valuable property in that it does not affect the transparency of the cytoplasm so that it is possible to examine clumps of cells in the smear as well as single discrete cells. The stain also provides information about the type of epithelial cells present in the smear. For example, squamous epithelial cells have a dense cyanophilic or eosinophilic cytoplasm, whereas glandular cells have very delicate cytoplasm. Cells which are highly keratinised (such as those found in invasive squamous carcinomas) have bright orange cytoplasm. Thus the colour and shape of the cells are important diagnostic features for the cytologist and these will only be preserved if the smears are properly prepared and fixed without drying.

Once the smear has been stained, it is dehydrated and mounted in Depex and a coverslip applied. It can now be examined under a microscope.

The primary screener examines the cells field by field – searching for the occasional abnormal cell amid hundreds of thousands of normal cells. If no abnormality is encountered, the primary screener may prepare and issue the report. If abnormality is suspected the smear is passed to a supervisor or the pathologist for a second opinion.

Screening is a labour-intensive task which requires a high level of skill and concentration. Each smear contains at least 300,000 cells and a primary screener in the UK is expected to examine 50 smears a day (more in other countries). It is hardly surprising that errors of diagnosis occur and false-negative reports are issued.

All laboratories have in place a quality control system which is designed to minimise the risk of overlooking an abnormal smear. This is achieved in most countries by the supervisor checking a random ten percent of negative smears, whereas in the UK it is achieved by 'rapid review' of all negative smears. Other quality control measures include retrospective review of smears of women who have a history of negative smears but who develop preinvasive or invasive cancer and cytological/histological/colposcopic correlation in women with an abnormal smear report.

The normal cells that can be recognised in a cervical smear are itemised below and include:

- *Squamous epithelial cells* from the ectocervical epithelium.
- *Endocervical cells* (also known as glandular or columnar cells) from the endocervical canal.
- *Immature metaplastic cells* from the transformation zone.
- *Epithelial and stromal cells* from the endometrial cavity, red blood cells and leucocytes.

In addition Doderlein bacilli, mucus strands and spermatozoa may be seen.

A number of specific infections can be identified with confidence, for example, *Candida* species, *Trichomonas vaginalis*, *Gardnerella vaginalis* (clue cells), actinomyces, HPV infection (koilocytes) and herpes genitalis. The smear also reflects the hormonal status of the patient in that smears taken from women with high levels of circulating oestrogen contain numerous large superficial squamous cells whereas smears taken from a postmenopausal women will be comprised of small squamous cells with an atrophic appearance, often described as 'parabasal cells' (Figures 9.5–9.11).

Neoplastic cells are recognised by virtue of their abnormal nuclei which are irregular in size and shape and their altered nucleo-cytoplasmic ratio. The nuclei may contain enlarged irregular nucleoli or mitotic figures, all of which are evidence of abnormal cell division which is a feature of malignancy. Several features distinguish smears containing cells from invasive squamous cancer of the cervix from smears containing cells from a precancerous lesion. Cells from invasive squamous cervical cancers are usually highly keratinised and vary greatly in shape and size. Moreover, smears from an invasive cancer are more likely to be heavily blood stained and contain polymorphs and necrotic cell debris. In contrast, precancerous cells are more uniform and the smears do not show a malignant diathesis. Cytologists can distinguish neoplastic cells from a squamous carcinoma from those

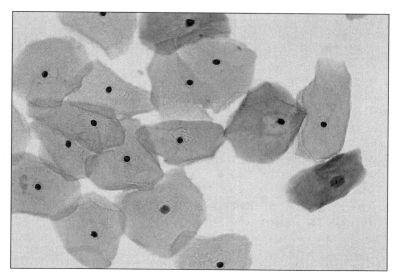

Figure 9.5 Normal squames in a cervical smear. Notice the low nucleo-cytoplasmic ratio and the delicate eosinophilic or cyanophilic staining of the cytoplasm.

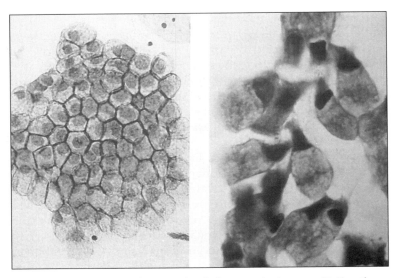

Figure 9.6 Normal endocervical cells in a cervical smear. Notice the columnar shape of the cells when they appear in palisade and the honeycomb pattern when the cells are seen *en face*.

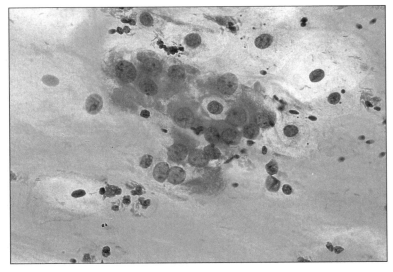

Figure 9.7 Immature metaplastic cells surrounded by mature squames. Note the difference in the nucleo-cytoplasmic ratio between the two cell types.

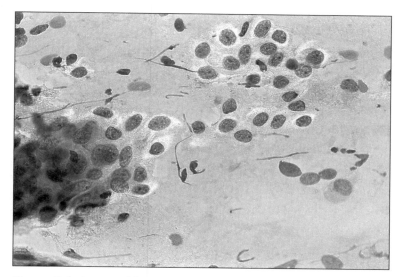

Figure 9.8 An atrophic pattern in a smear from a postmenopausal woman. These smears often contain scanty small parabasal cells which usually show marked inflammatory degenerative changes.

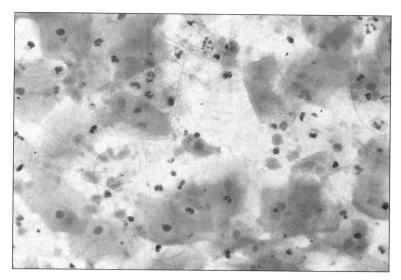

Figure 9.9 Trichomonads in a cervical smear. They appear as slate grey bodies.

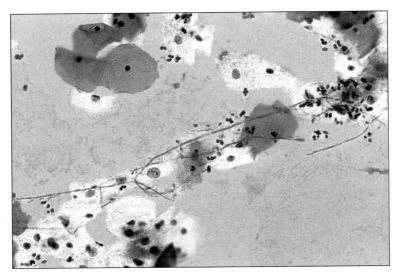

Figure 9.10 *Candida* spores and hyphae in a cervical smear.

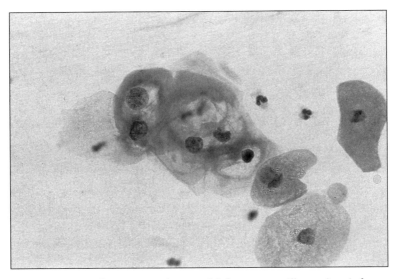

Figure 9.11 Koilocytes consistent with human papillomavirus infection. Note the slight nuclear enlargement and irregularity which amounts to 'borderline nuclear change'.

from adenocarcinoma and they can even pick up clues from the smear as to whether the adenocarcinoma is endocervical or endometrial in origin (Figures 9.12–9.14).

The smear report

A smear report should be provided in narrative form and should contain the following information:

1 Whether the smear is adequate for reporting.
2 A description of the cells seen and the histological lesion predicted.
3 Management guidelines.

The terminology used to report cervical smears in the UK is shown in Table 9.3. An equivalent terminology (the Bethesda system) in use in the USA and some European countries is shown in Table 9.4. The Bethesda system differs from the UK system in that it introduces several new categories of lesion, namely high-grade and low-grade squamous intraepithelial lesions (HSIL and LSIL) and atypical squamous (or glandular) epithelial lesion of unknown significance (ASCUS or AGUS). These two categories roughly equate to the CIN nomencla-

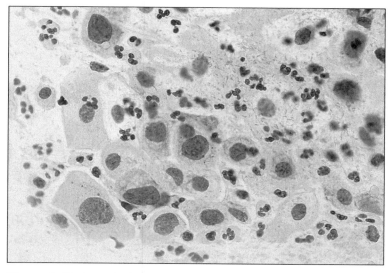

Figure 9.12 A cervical smear containing squamous cells showing severe dyskaryosis consistent with CIN 3. Note abnormal nucleo-cytoplasmic ratio and variation in nuclear size and shape.

Table 9.3 Interpretation of smear results (based on terminology recommended by the British Society for Clinical Cytology)

Cytology report	Explanation	Action
Inadequate	Insufficient cellular material Inadequate fixation Smear consisting mainly of blood or inflammatory exudate Little or no material to suggest that the transformation zone has been sampled	Repeat smear
Negative	Normal Includes simple inflammatory changes including a mild polymorph exudate	Routine recall
Borderline changes with or without HPV change	Cellular appearances that cannot be described as normal Smears in which there is doubt as to whether the nuclear changes are inflammatory or dyskaryosis	Repeat smear at six months Consider for colposcopy if changes persist
Mild dyskaryosis with or without HPV change	Cellular appearances consistent with origin from CIN (mild dysplasia)	Repeat smear at six months Consider for colposcopy if changes persist
Moderate dyskaryosis with or without HPV change	Cellular appearances consistent with origin from CIN 2 (moderate dysplasia)	Refer for colposcopy
Severe dyskaryosis with or without HPV change	Cellular appearances consistent with origin from CIN 3 (severe dysplasia/carcinoma *in situ*)	Refer for colposcopy
Severe dyskaryosis/ ? invasive carcinoma	Cellular appearances consistent with origin from CIN 3, but with additional features which suggest the possibility of invasive cancer	Refer for colposcopy
Glandular neoplasia or suspicion of glandular	Cellular appearances suggesting pre-cancer or cancer in the cervical canal or the endometrium	Refer for colposcopy

Source: Austoker, J. and McPherson, A. (1992) *Practical Guides for General Practice (14): Cervical Screening.* Oxford: Cancer Research Campaign/Oxford Medical Publications

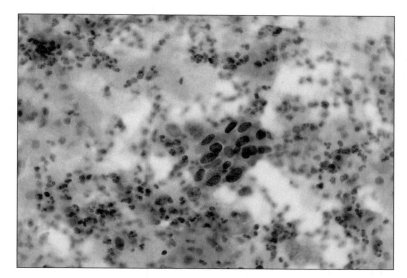

Figure 9.13 Severe dyskaryosis in a cervical smear. The nuclear pleo-morphism, numerous polymorphs and blood-stained background suggest invasive cancer rather than CIN.

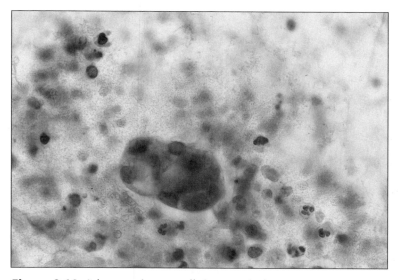

Figure 9.14 Adenocarcinoma cells in a cervical smear.

Table 9.4 Bethesda system

Adequacy of the specimen
Satisfactory for evaluation
Satisfactory for evaluation but limited by . . . (specify reason)
Unsatisfactory for evaluation . . . (specify reason)

General categorisation (optional)
Within normal limits
Benign cellular changes: see descriptive diagnosis
Epithelial cell abnormality: see descriptive diagnosis

Descriptive diagnoses
Benign cellular changes:
    INFECTION
    Trichomonas vaginalis
    Fungal organisms morphologically consistent with *Candida* spp.
    Predominance of coccobacilli consistent with shift in vaginal flora
    Bacteria morphologically consistent with *Actinomyces* spp.
    Cellular changes associated with herpes simplex virus
    Other[a]
    REACTIVE CHANGES
    Reactive cellular changes associated with:
        inflammation (includes typical repair)
        atrophy with inflammation ('atrophic vaginitis')
        radiation
        intrauterine contraceptive device
        other

Epithelial cell abnormalities
    SQUAMOUS CELL
    Atypical squamous cells of undetermined significance: qualify
    Low-grade squamous intraepithelial lesion (LSIL) encompassing: HPV[a], mild
        dysplasia/CIN 1
    High-grade squamous intraepithelial lesion (HSIL) encompassing: moderate
        and severe dysplasia, CIS/CIN 2 and CIN 3
    GLANDULAR CELL
    Endometrial cells, cytologically benign in a postmenopausal woman
    Atypical glandular cells of undetermined significance: qualify[b]
    Endocervical adenocarcinoma
    Endometrial adenocarcinoma
    Extrauterine adenocarcinoma
    Adenocarcinoma, not otherwise specified

Other malignant neoplasms: specify

Hormonal evaluation (applies to vaginal smears only)
    Hormonal pattern compatible with age and history
    Hormonal pattern incompatible with age and history: specify
    Hormonal evaluation not possible due to: specify

[a] Cellular changes of human papillomavirus (HPV) (previously termed koilocytosis, koilocytis atypia and condylomatous atypia) are included in the category LSIL
[b] Atypical squamous or glandular cells of undetermined significance should be further qualified, if possible, as to whether a premalignant/malignant process is favoured

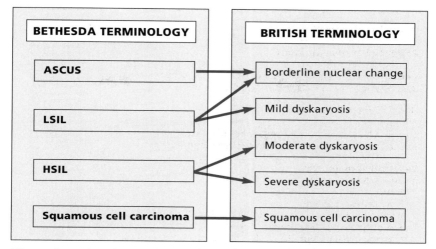

Figure 9.15 Correlation between UK and Bethesda reporting systems: squamous epithelial cell abnormalities.

ture and the borderline lesions used in the UK. A major point of difference, however, is that the Bethesda system classifies the cytological changes consistent with HPV infection as LSIL whereas in the UK, koilocytes showing a slight nuclear atypia due to HPV infection, are considered to show borderline changes (Figure 9.15).

Interpretation of the cervical smear report

THE UNSATISFACTORY CERVICAL SMEAR

Smears may be unsatisfactory for five reasons (Figures 9.16 and 9.17).
1 They may be too thickly spread to allow inspection of the cells or too scanty and air-dried due to faulty smear-taking procedure (the latter is not uncommon in smears from postmenopausal women).
2 The relevant epithelial cells may be obscured by polymorphs if there is a severe cervicitis.
3 A postcoital smear may contain so many spermatozoa that they obscure the epithelial cells.
4 Red blood cells may obscure the epithelial cells on the slide (this is particularly common in smears taken at the onset or during menstruation or in invasive cancer).
5 Cell morphology may be poorly displayed due to cytolysis (this is most likely to occur when smears are taken in the late secretory phase of the cycle or in early pregnancy).

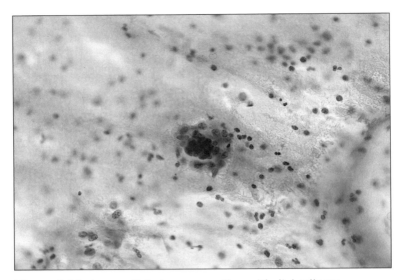

Figure 9.16 An unsatisfactory smear: the epithelial cells are obscured by red blood cells.

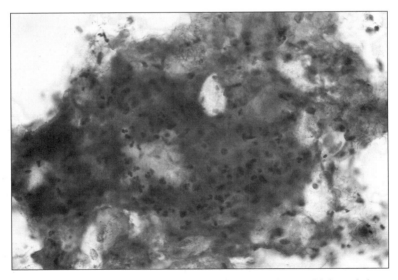

Figure 9.17 An unsatisfactory smear: the smear is too thick and the morphology of the squamous cells cannot be visualised.

Many unsatisfactory smears can be avoided by good smear-taking technique and ensuring the smear is taken mid-cycle. It is good practice for cytology laboratories to report the individual 'unsatisfactory smear rate' at regular intervals to the clinicians sending smears to the laboratory for analysis. The unsatisfactory smear rate should not exceed 7%.

THE SATISFACTORY SMEAR

A satisfactory smear contains numerous epithelial cells which are evenly spread and clearly displayed. It should also contain evidence of transformation zone sampling. Thus it should contain one or more of the following elements in addition to the squamous epithelial cells:

1 Endocervical (glandular cells).
2 Immature metaplastic cells.
3 Mucus strands.

In some centres the presence of one or more of these components is recorded in the smear report.

There are those who consider a smear to be inadequate and unsuitable for assessment if it does not contain endocervical cells or immature metaplastic cells but opinion is divided on this issue. It has been shown that CIN can be detected just as efficiently in smears without endocervical cells as in smears with them, so that absence of endocervical cells can hardly be construed as evidence of an unsatisfactory smear or as an indicator of need for a repeat smear.

According to the Bethesda system of reporting cervical smears, smears which appear to be satisfactory in every other way but lack endocervical cells should be reported as 'suboptimal'. This practice is strongly discouraged in the UK for legal reasons.

Negative

The majority of smears are reported as negative, indicating that they contain no evidence of malignancy. However, other information about the smear which may be useful for the clinician in his or her management of the patient should be reported. This includes information about specific infection, such as *Trichomonas*, or the presence of endometrial cells in a smear from a postmenopausal woman.

Mild, moderate and severe dyskaryosis

Smears containing cells showing varying degrees of dyskaryosis (nuclear abnormality) indicate the presence of a focus of intraepithelial neoplasia in the cervix. A mild degree of dyskaryosis is suggestive of CIN 1, whereas moderate and severe dyskaryosis are suggestive of CIN 2 and CIN 3, respectively. It is not uncommon for a cytologist to find both mild and moderately dyskaryotic cells in the smear, reflecting foci of both CIN 1 and CIN 2 in the cervix. It is usual to report the most severe degree of dyskaryosis in the smear.

Severe dyskaryosis/invasive squamous carcinoma

It should be remembered that cytology involves the examination of cells shed from the *surface* layers of the epithelium lining the ecto- and endocervix and a definitive diagnosis of actual invasion of the sub-epithelial connective tissue by neoplastic cells cannot be made on the smear. Thus, the smear report can only provide a provisional diagnosis which requires confirmation by biopsy. Despite this limitation, experienced cytopathologists can be remarkably accurate in their prediction as to whether a lesion is invasive or intraepithelial and a cytodiagnosis of possible invasion should not be ignored. The number of abnormal cells in a smear gives no indication of the size or the location of the lesion and colposcopy is essential in such cases.

Cytologists have to be aware of the effect of radiotherapy or cyto-toxic drug therapy on the cervical epithelium. These forms of therapy produce changes very similar to dyskaryosis and may lead to misinter-pretation of the smear. Smears taken within three months of laser ablation or biopsy often contain atypical cells. It is important for the cytologist to be given a full clinical history to minimise the risk of such mistakes. Women on hormone replacement therapy often have a proliferative pattern with abundant endocervical cells, which can be misleading unless the clinical history is known.

Glandular neoplasia

Endocervical adenocarcinoma accounts for 20% of cases of cervical cancer and should be suspected in those cases where the smear contains numerous endocervical cells with slightly enlarged nuclei showing anisonucleosis. The glandular cells shed from a well-differen-tiated adenocarcinoma and adenocarcinoma *in situ* tend to be arranged in papillary fronds or rosettes, whereas less well-differentiated tumours shed dense clumps of tumour cells. Cytologists can sometimes distin-guish cells shed from an endometrial or ovarian cancer from those of an endocervical adenocarcinoma, as the former are often scanty and poorly preserved.

Nuclear changes bordering on dyskaryosis

There is always a small number of cases where the cytologist finds it difficult to decide whether the nuclear changes in the epithelial cells can be attributed to an inflammatory response or to neoplasia. In such cases a report of 'borderline changes' is given and the patient is kept under cytological surveillance. This is a common problem in smears containing evidence of HPV infection, as the koilocytes often have slightly abnormal nuclei (Figure 9.11). It is also a problem after radiotherapy and sometimes in atrophic smears.

Studies have shown that the proportion of cases reported as showing mild dyskaryosis/borderline changes varies from laboratory to laboratory. To overcome this problem a single management system (repeat in six months) is advocated for women whose smears show these changes. After two or more borderline smears colposcopy is advised.

The weakness of this management scheme is that it puts an unnecessary strain on the patient and the clinical resources as no significant pathology is found at colposcopy in the majority of cases. Clearly, unrestricted use of the borderline category could overwhelm the screening system and careful evaluation of smears is needed to ensure optimal use of resources.

Management

The management of women with an abnormal smear is controversial and is individual to the clinician and the patient. The main aim of management is to ensure that all women with an abnormal smear receive appropriate treatment and follow-up. It is important to ensure that facilities are available for this and expert colposcopic opinion can be provided without delay. The management plan adopted at St Mary's Hospital in London is shown in Figure 9.18. Certain principles should be adhered to:

1 Borderline changes (including HPV changes) or mild dyskaryosis in a young woman below the age of 35 can be managed conservatively by a repeat smear in the first instance, whereas mild dyskaryosis in an older woman is an indication for colposcopy and biopsy.

2 Moderate or severe dyskaryosis at any age is an indication for colposcopy.

3 If there is a discrepancy between the cytology, colposcopy and biopsy findings, the results should be reviewed and action taken on the basis of the review.

4 Recurrent or persistent mild dyskaryosis or borderline change or two consecutive unsatisfactory smears are indications for further investigation by colposcopy.

5 The patient's age, clinical history and level of compliance must always be considered when planning management.

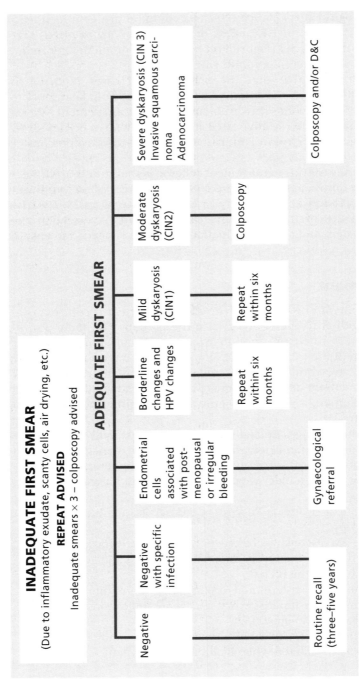

Figure 9.18 Protocol for the management of smears. The guidelines apply to women under the age of 35. Older women with abnormal smear merit closer surveillance or earlier referral for colposcopy due to their increased risk of cervical cancer. Severe dyskaryosis at any stage merits immediate referral to colposcopy as does any clinical indication of carcinoma.

HYSTERECTOMY FOLLOWING CIN

Vaginal vault smears are valuable in the follow-up of women who have had CIN managed by hysterectomy rather than by local treatment. Although hysterectomy is not infrequently the treatment of choice in cases of invasive cervical cancer, it is rarely indicated for the treatment of CIN. It has a place, however, in biopsy where histological examination of the excision margins indicates incomplete removal of CIN. Hysterectomy may also be appropriate in those cases where follow-up cytology suggests residual or recurrent CIN after local treatment. In these cases, vault smears should be taken at regular intervals to ensure that the CIN lesion has been completely removed and to detect early recurrence in the vagina or vulva. Any suggestion of field change in the vagina or vulva should be followed by biopsy before the start of treatment. Vault smears and vaginal smears after hysterectomy for CIN or invasive cervical cancer can sometimes be difficult to interpret microscopically, as radiotherapy changes or granulation tissue or even prolapsed fallopian tube tissue can mimic neoplasia in the smears.

The future of cervical cytology

There is little doubt that a well-organised cervical screening programme can be an effective method of reducing mortality and morbidity from cervical cancer. However, the programme is costly and, in countries without a nationally funded programme, it is the women least at risk who can afford a regular smear test. Moreover, there is a high false-negative rate associated with the Papanicolaou test, due in part to poor smear-taking but also due to errors of reporting. The challenge, therefore, is to develop a more cost-effective and more accurate method of screening. Two approaches to screening are under investigation, namely testing for HPV infection and automated analysis of cervical smears.

SCREENING FOR HPV INFECTION

Within the last 15 years evidence has accumulated which indicates that HPV plays a role in the development of most cervical cancers. The evidence is drawn from studies of the prevalence of DNA sequences from oncogenic HPV strains (HPV 16, 18 and 32) in cancerous and precancerous cervical lesions and from demonstration of the transforming properties of these cancer-associated HPV strains *in vitro* and in experimental animals. Moreover, prospective studies indicate that women who harbour HPV 16 in the cervical epithelium may have a greater risk of developing CIN 3 than women who are HPV-negative.

These observations have led to the suggestion that HPV testing could be used as a screening tool to identify women who are at greatest risk of developing cancer.

Several studies have been carried out since 1992 to determine the value of such a screening system. The molecular techniques most favoured for virus detection are the polymerase chain reaction (PCR), which is a highly sensitive method of detecting HPV sequences, or hybrid capture, which permits quantification of HPV DNA. Unfortunately, both approaches have their drawbacks. For example, although PCR is highly-sensitive, it must be carried out under conditions of the utmost stringency to minimise the risk of contamination. In addition, the interpretation of the results of the test is largely subjective. Hybrid capture is limited by the number of virus types which can be identified in a single test and there would always be a small group of women at risk of developing cervical cancers which would be missed by the test. For these reasons, HPV screening for cervical cancer has not been adopted and further research is needed to establish a reliable test.

AUTOMATED ANALYSIS OF CERVICAL SMEARS

There have been several occasions recently both in the UK and the USA when laboratories have been severely criticised by the press and public for failing to provide a reliable cytodiagnostic service. Errors of reporting cervical smears have put women's lives at risk and have led to loss of confidence in the cervical screening programme. The response to this unfortunate situation has been to examine alternative methods of screening which might offer a higher degree of accuracy and reliability of performance.

One method which is currently under intense investigation is the automated analysis of cervical smears. A model automated system should meet the following specifications:

1 The system should detect all samples that contain neoplastic cells.
2 The system should not flag 'false alarms' on normal cells.
3 The system should not render the smear unsuitable for classical microscope review.
4 The results should be reproducible.
5 The system should identify inadequate smears.
6 The system should operate cost effectively.

It is worth noting that the need to detect infectious organisms and hormonal discrepancy is not a requirement of a model screening system. At present there is no stand-alone automated system which meets these requirements. However, several interactive automated systems have been approved by the Federal Food and Drug Agency in the USA for quality control purposes and are now commercially available. One of these systems, the PAPNET system, is currently under evaluation in the UK as a primary screening tool.

The PAPNET automated system for the analysis of cervical smears was developed by Neuromedical Systems Inc., Suffern, New York, USA and is designed to increase the accuracy of reporting conventionally-prepared cervical smears without introducing any new source of risk. It is an interactive system based on neural network technology, which is a branch of artificial intelligence ideally suited for recognising patterns in natural scenes. Papanicolaou-stained smears are scanned by an electronic camera which extracts the 128 most abnormal cells in the smear and records them on compact disc. The images are examined by the cytologist at a PAPNET review station who triages them as 'normal' or 'review'. Smears identified as normal are not examined further. Smears coded for review are examined in the conventional way in the light microscope. Thus, the PAPNET system does not attempt to diagnose the smear: rather, it facilitates analysis by retaining the subjective and subtle diagnostic interpretation that only the human intellect can provide. Several studies have shown that the PAPNET system can reduce the false-negative rate to less than three percent (Figure 9.19).

The effectiveness of the PAPNET system for primary screening is currently being investigated in the UK. The National Health Service is currently funding a trial of the PAPNET system which involves comparison of the results of PAPNET analysis with conventional microscopy of the same smears. Five laboratories are participating, each contributing 4000 consecutive smears (total 20,000). The trial is co-ordinated by the Department of Cytopathology at St Mary's Hospital in London.

Data from the project will be used to assess the likely effects of automation-assisted screening on laboratory performance and costs. A favourable outcome may well change the face of cytology screening in the years to come.

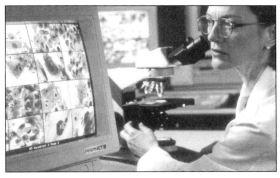

Figure 9.19 The PAPNET system: the cytologist makes the decision as to whether this smear needs further investigation by light microscopy after she has examined the cells shown in the 128 tiles displayed on the monitor.

Suggested references for further reading

Buckley, C.H. and Fox, H. (1998) *Biopsy Pathology of the Endometrium,* 2nd ed. London: Chapman and Hall

Buntinx, F. and Brouwers, M. (1996) Relation between sampling device and detection of abnormality in cervical smears; a meta-analysis of randomised and quasi randomised studies. *BMJ* **313**, 1285–90

Coleman, D.V. (1995) 'Gynecological cytopathology' in H. Fox (Ed.) *Haines and Taylor: Obstetrical and Gynecological Pathology,* 4th ed., pp. 1393–436. Edinburgh: Churchill Livingstone

Coleman, D.V. and Evans D.M.D. (1988) *Biopsy Pathology and Cytology of the Cervix.* London: Chapman and Hall

Coleman, D.V., Day, N., Douglas, G. *et al.* (1993) European Guidelines for Quality Assurance in Cervical Cancer Screening. *Eur J Cancer* **29A** (suppl. 4), S1–S38

Fox, H. (Ed.) (1995) *Haines and Taylor: Obstetrical and Gynaecological Pathology,* 4th ed. Edinburgh: Churchill Livingstone

Fox, H. (1997) *Pathology of the Placenta,* 2nd ed. London: WB Saunders

Fu, Y.S. and Reagan, J.W. (1989) *Pathology of the Uterine Cervix, Vagina and Vulva.* Philadelphia: WB Saunders

Holland, W.W. and Stewart, S. (1990) 'Screening in adult women' in *Screening in Health Care,* pp. 155–71. London: Nuffield Provincial Hospitals Trust

Kurman, R.J. (Ed.) (1994) *Blaustein's Pathology of the Female Genital Tract,* 4th ed. New York: Springer Verlag

Mazur, M.T. and Kurman, R.J. (1994) *Diagnosis of Endometrial Biopsies and Curettings.* New York: Springer Verlag

National Health Service Cervical Screening Programme (1997) I.D. Duncan (Ed.) *Guidelines for Clinical Practice and Programme Management* (2nd ed.) Sheffield: NHSCSP

Ridley, C.M. and Neill, S. (1998) *The Vulva,* 2nd ed. Oxford: Blackwell Science

Russell, P. and Farnworth, A. (1997) *Surgical Pathology of the Ovaries,* 2nd ed. Edinburgh: Churchill Livingstone

Wilkinson, E.J. (Ed.) (1987) *Pathology of the Vulva and Vagina.* Edinburgh: Churchill Livingstone

Zaino, R.J. (1996) *Interpretation of Endometrial Biopsies and Curettings.* Philadelphia, Lipincott-Raven

Index

A

abdominal pregnancy 128
Addison's disease 94
adenoacanthoma, endometrium 63
adenocarcinoma
  Bartholin's gland 17
  cervix, *see* cervical carcinoma,
    glandular
  endocervical 41
  endometrium 61–5
  enteric 42
  fallopian tube 83–4, 85
  mesonephric 42
  ovarian 96, 102–3
  Paget's disease of vulva and 10
  vulvar 10
  see also clear-cell adenocarcinoma;
    endometrioid adenocarcinoma;
    serous adenocarcinoma
adenocarcinoma *in situ*
  arising in endometriosis 125
  cervix 40–1, 164
  fallopian tube 84, 85
adenoid cystic adenocarcinoma,
  Bartholin's gland 17
adenomatoid tumour
  fallopian tube 83
  myometrium 74–5
adenomyoma 71
adenomyosis 71, 72
adenosarcoma, endometrium 68
adenosis, vaginal 20–1
adenosquamous carcinoma
  cervix 42–3
  endometrium 65–6
adhesions
  intrauterine 55
  peri-ovarian 87, 88
adnexal (skin appendage) neoplasms,
  malignant 16
alpha-fetoprotein (AFP) 115, 116
androblastoma 110–3
androstenedione 62, 91

Asherman's syndrome 55
automated analysis, cervical smears
  168–9
Aylesbury spatula 149
Ayres spatula 149

B

bacterial vaginosis 19
Bartholin's gland
  carcinoma 17
  duct cysts 11
basal cell carcinoma, vulva 16
basal cell naevus syndrome 109
basal cell papillomas, vulva 12
Bethesda system 157, 160, 171, 173
Bowen's disease, Bowenoid papulosis,
  see vulvar intraepithelial neoplasia
BRCA-1, BRCA-2 genes 103
Brenner tumours 95, 100, 101
  malignant 100, 101, 102

C

Call–Exner bodies 106, 107
Calymmatobacterium granulomatis 3
candidiasis (*Candida*) 19–20
  in cervical smears 153, 159
carcinoid tumours, ovarian 118–20
carcinosarcoma, endometrium 68, 69
cervical carcinoma
  diagnosis 145
  follow-up 145–50, 167
  glandular (adenocarcinoma) 39, 41–2
    cervical smear 157, 159, 164
  invasive squamous cell 31–3, 35–6,
    37–9
    aetiology 32–3
    cervical smear 153, 164
  microinvasive (stage Ia invasive) 36–7
  mixed pattern 42–3
  screening 143–5
  small cell 43
cervical cytology, *see* cervical smear

cervical glandular intraepithelial
neoplasia (CGIN, GIN) 40
cervical intraepithelial neoplasia (CIN)
6, 31–2, 33–6
aetiological factors 32–3
cervical smears 153, 157, 161, 163–4
follow-up 145–6, 168
grade 1 (CIN 1) 33, 34
grade 2 (CIN 2) 33, 34
grade 3 (CIN 3) 33, 35
HPV infections and 31
cervical smear 143–69
automated analysis 169–70
Bethesda system 157, 160, 161, 163
borderline nuclear changes 164–5
dyskariosis 159, 163–4, 165
future prospects 167–9
glandular neoplasia 164
indications 143–6
interpretation of report 161–5
invasive squamous carcinoma 153,
164
management of abnormal 165–7
negative 163
preparation/interpretation 161–7
reports 167–71
satisfactory 173–5
specimen collection 146–51
combined scrape/brush technique
150
endocervical brush 148, 149–51
sampling devices 149, 151
scrape technique 146–9
suboptimal 163
UK system 157, 158, 161
unsatisfactory 161–3
cervicitis 26–30
follicular 28, 29
infective 27–30
non-infective 27
cervix 25–43
bacterial infections 28–9
biopsy 145, 146
condylomata (warts) 28, 31
ectopy/ectropion 25
glandular neoplasia 39–42, 164
inflammatory disease 26–30
neoplasms 31–43
physiological changes 25–6
polyps 30
in pregnancy 26
protozoal infections 29–30
squamous neoplasia 31–3
strawberry 29–30
viral infections 28
chancre, syphilitic 5, 29
chancroid 5
Chlamydia trachomatis infections 5, 28,

29, 78
chorangioma 139–141
chorioamnionitis 139
choriocarcinoma 132–5
hydatidiform mole and 130, 132, 133
ovary 115
CIN, *see* cervical intraepithelial neoplasia
clear-cell adenocarcinoma
arising in endometriosis 125
cervix 41–2
endometrium 64, 65
ovary 102–3
vagina 23
clear-cell tumours, ovary 95, 102
clue cells 153
colposcopy 145, 146, 165
condylomata, flat 6, 28, 31
condylomata acuminata
cervix 28, 31
vulva 4–6
condylomata lata 4, 20
contraceptive methods, cervical
neoplasia and 32
corpus luteum cysts 89, 90
cytotoxic drug therapy, cervical cytology
and 164

D

decubital ulceration, cervix 27
dermatological disorders 1–3
dermoids (mature cystic teratomas) 83,
117–8
dichorionic-diamniotic pregnancy 141–2
diethylstilboestrol (DES) 21, 23
Donovan bodies 3
dysgerminoma 114, 115

E

ectopic pregnancy 127–8
embryonal rhabdomyosarcoma, vaginal
24
endocervical adenocarcinoma 41
endocervical brush 148, 149–51
endocervical cells, cervical smear 152,
154, 163
endodermal sinus tumours 115–16
endometrial cells, cervical smear 152
endometrial hyperplasia 51, 57–61, 91
atypical 58, 59–61, 65
complex 59, 60
simple (cystic glandular) 58–9
endometrial stromal metaplasia 55
endometrial stromal sarcoma 66–7
endometrioid adenocarcinoma
arising in endometriosis 125
cervix 42
endometrium 62–3, 64
ovary 99–100, 102–3

endometrioid tumours, ovary 95,
  99–100
endometriosis 122–5
  extraovarian pelvic 125
  ovarian 123–5
endometritis 52–5
  active chronic 53, 54
  acute 53, 55
  chronic granulomatous 53–55
  chronic non-granulomatous 53
  histiocytic/xanthomatous 53
  infective 52–5
  non-infective 52
endometrium 45–69
  adenocarcinoma 61–5
  atrophy 48, 49
  functional abnormalities 50–2
  histology 45–9
  inflammation/infection 52–5
  malignant epithelial tumours 61–6
  menstrual cycle changes 45–8
  metaplasia 55, 56
  mixed tumours 68, 69
  polyps 55–7
  in postmenopausal women 48, 49, 50
  proliferative phase 45, 48
  secretory phase 46–8
  senile cystic change 49
endosalpingiosis 105
  atypical 105
endosalpingitis 77, 78–80
epidermoid cysts 11
epithelial inclusion cysts, ovary 87–8, 95
erythroplasia of Queyrat, *see* vulvar
  intraepithelial neoplasia

F

fallopian tube 77–85
  carcinoma 82, 83–4, 85
  cysts 81–2
  ectopic pregnancy 127–8
  inflammation 77–81
  rupture 128
  tumours 82–4
fetus
  growth retardation 136, 138, 139,
    140
  hypoxia 136, 140
  intrauterine death 136, 140
fibrin, perivillous deposition 136, 137
fibroepitheliomatous polyps, vulva 12
fibroids (leiomyomas), uterine 71–4
fibromas, ovarian 109–10
fibrothecoma 109
follicle stimulating hormone (FSH) 91
follicular cysts 88–9

G

Gardnerella vaginalis 18, 153
germ cell tumours 114–19
glandular cells, cervical smear 152
gonadotrophin-resistant ovary syndrome
  93–4
gonorrhoea (*Neisseria gonorrhoeae*) 20,
  29, 53, 78
Gorlin's syndrome 109
granuloma inguinale 3
granulosa cell tumours
  adult type 106–8
  juvenile 108
growth retardation, fetal 136, 138, 139,
  140
gynandroblastoma 113

H

haemangioma, placental 139–41
Haemophilus ducreyi 4
haemorrhage
  in endometriosis 123
  ovarian 94
herpes simplex virus infections 3, 29
heterologous elements, endometrial
  tumours 68, 69
hidradenomas, vulvar 12
hormone replacement therapy 61–2,
  164
  see also oestrogen
HPV, *see* human papillomavirus
human chorionic gonadotrophin (hCG)
  89, 131
human papillomavirus (HPV)
  cervical infection 29, 32
  cervical neoplasia and 31, 33, 35, 39
  in cervical smears 153, 156, 161, 165
  screening for 167–8
  subclinical infection 6
  vulvar infection 3, 4–6
  vulvar neoplasia and 6, 14
hybrid capture 168
hydatidiform mole 128–32, 133
  complete 128–31
  invasive 132
  partial 131–2
hydatid of Morgagni 82
hydrosalpinx 79
  follicular 79
hypercalcaemia 121
hysterectomy, cytological follow-up
  151, 167

I

ichthyosis uteri 55, 66
immature metaplastic cells, cervical
  smear 152, 154, 163

inclusion cysts, ovarian 87–8, 95
infections
  in cervical smears 153, 155, 156
  cervix 27–30
  endometrium 52–5
  ovary 87, 88
  placenta 139
  vagina 19–20
  vulva 3–4
intrauterine contraceptive device (IUCD)
  127

K

K cells (endometrial lymphocytes) 48,
  52
keratoacanthomas 12
koilocytes 5, 31
  in cervical smears 153, 156, 165
Krukenberg tumour 123

L

laser ablation, cervical cytology after
  164
leiomyomas 71–4
  benign metastasising 74
  cellular 72
  epithelioid 73
  neurilemmoma-like 72–3
  parasitic 72
  'red degeneration' 73
  symplastic 73
  with tubules 73
leiomyomatosis
  disseminated peritoneal 74
  intravenous 73–4
leiomyosarcoma 75
Leydig cell neoplasms 110–11
lichen sclerosus 1–3, 14
lichen simplex 1, 2
lipomas 83
luteal phase insufficiency 50–1
luteinised unruptured follicle syndrome
  94
luteinising hormone (LH) 91
luteoma, pregnancy 92
lymphocytes, endometrial 48, 52
lymphogranuloma venereum 4

M

mamillary body 117
Meig's syndrome 109
melanoma, malignant 16
menopause, premature 93
menstrual cycle, endometrial histology
  45–7
menstruation, retrograde 123
mesonephric cysts 10–11, 81–2

metastatic tumours
  ovary 121–2
  vulva 17
mixed Müllerian tumours, endometrium
  68
monochorionic diamniotic pregnancy
  141, 142
monochorionic monoamniotic pregnancy 141, 142
mucinous adenocarcinoma 98, 99,
  102–3
mucinous cystadenoma 97–8
mucinous tumours, ovary 95, 97–9
  of borderline malignancy 104–5
mucous cysts, vulva 11
myometrium 71–5
  benign tumours 71–5
  malignant neoplasms 75

N

Nabothian follicles 25
Neisseria gonorrhoeae (gonorrhoea) 20,
  28, 53, 78

O

obesity, endometrial adenocarcinoma
  and 61, 62
oedema, massive, of ovary 91–2
oestrogen
  endometrial adenocarcinoma and
    61–2
  endometrial effects 50, 51
  endometrial hyperplasia and 59
  -secreting ovarian tumours 62, 107
  unopposed therapy 51, 59, 62
oestrone 62, 91
oophoritis, autoimmune 94
oral contraceptive pill 32, 52
ovarian cancer genes 103
ovarian cysts
  derived from surface epithelium 87–8
  endometriotic 123–4, 125
    follicular 88–9
  non-neoplastic 87–91
  torsion 90
ovarian failure, premature 93–4
ovarian hyperstimulation syndrome
  89–90
ovarian tumours 94–122
  adenocarcinoma 96, 102–3
  epithelial 94–105
    benign/malignant 95–6
    of borderline malignancy 96, 103–5
  germ cell 114–19
  metastatic 121–2
  miscellaneous 119–21
  of non-specialised ovarian tissue 119
  oestrogen-secreting 62, 107

sex cord stromal 105–113
see also specific types
ovary 87–125
    endometriosis 123–5
    gonadotrophin-resistant 93–4
    haemorrhage 94
    infections 87, 88
    inflammation 87
    massive oedema 91–2
    stromal hyperplasia/hyperthecosis 91
ovulation 46
    failure 50–1

P

p53 tumour suppressor gene 33
Paget's disease, vulva 10
Papanicolaou (Pap) test, *see* cervical
    smear
Papanicolaou stain 151–2
papillary serous adenocarcinoma, *see*
    serous adenocarcinoma (papillary)
PAPNET system 169
paramesonephric cysts 81–2
pelvic abscess 79
pelvic inflammatory disease (PID) 77
perioophoritis 86, 87
peritoneal cysts, vulva 10–11
peritonitis 78, 79
perivillous fibrin deposition 136, 137
persistent trophoblastic disease 131, 132
Peutz–Jeghers syndrome 113
placenta 134–142
    circummarginate 134–5
    circumvallate 134–5
    developmental abnormalities 134–5
    extrachorialis 134, 135
    gross lesions 136–7
    infarction 136–7
    infections 139
    insufficiency 137–8
    non-trophoblastic tumours 139–41
    in twin pregnancy 139–40
placental site trophoblastic tumour 134,
    135
polycystic ovary syndrome (PCOS) 62,
    90–91
polyhydramnios 140
polymerase chain reaction (PCR) 168
polymorphonuclear leucocytes, endome-
    trial 48, 52, 53
posterior fornix aspiration 151
postmenopausal women
    cervical smears 153, 155
    endometrial histology 48, 49, 50
pre-decidual cells 48
pre-eclampsia 137, 138
pregnancy
    cervix in 26

ectopic 127–8
    luteoma 92
    related abnormalities 127–42
premature rupture of membranes 139
preterm labour 139
progesterone, endometrial histology and
    50–1
progestogens, endometrial effects 51–2
prolapse, uterine 27
pseudomyxoma peritonei 98–9
pyosalpinx 79

Q

quality control, cervical cytology 152

R

radiotherapy, cervical cytology and 164
Reinke's crystals 110
retention cysts, cervix 25
Rokitansky's tubercle 117

S

salpingitis 77–81
    ascending infection 77, 78–80
    blood-borne infection 77, 81
    follicular 79
    isthmica nodosa 80
    lymphatic infection 77, 80
sarcoma botryoides 24
Schiller–Duval bodies 116
schistosomiasis 30
screening
    cervical cancer 143–5
    HPV infection 167–8
seborrhoeic keratoses, vulva 12
serous adenocarcinoma (papillary)
    cervix 42
    endometrium 63–4
    ovary 97, 102–3
serous cystadenofibroma 97
serous cystadenomas, ovary 88, 96
serous inclusion cysts, ovarian 87–8
serous tumours, ovary 95, 96–7, 102
    of borderline malignancy 104, 105
Sertoli cell tumours 110
Sertoli–Leydig cell tumours 111–13
sex cord stromal tumours 105–13
sex cord tumour with annular tubules
    113
sexually transmitted infections 3–4,
    19–20, 32–3
sexual partners, number of 32
signet-ring cells 123
skin appendage neoplasms, malignant
    16
skin tags, vulva 12

small cell carcinoma
  cervix 43
  ovary 121
smoking, cigarette 6, 32
spiral arteries 138
spirochaetal infections (syphilis) 4, 20, 29
squamous cell carcinoma
  Bartholin's gland 17
  cervix, *see* cervical carcinoma, invasive squamous cell
  endometrium 66
  vagina 22
  vulva 9, 13–15
squamous epithelial cells, cervical smear 152
squamous hyperplasia, vulva 1, 14
squamous metaplasia
  cervix 25
  endometrium 55, 56, 63
squamous papillomas, vulva 12
steroid cell tumours, ovary 119–21
strumal carcinoid, ovarian 120
struma ovarii 118–120
sweat gland tumours 12
syphilis (spirochaetal infections) 4, 20, 29

T
teratomas 114, 116–20
  immature 117, 118, 119
  malignant 117, 118
  mature 117
  mature cystic (dermoids) 83, 117–18
  monophyletic 116–17, 118–19
thecomas 109
thyroid tissue, ovarian 118, 119–20
transformation zone, cervical 25, 32
trichomoniasis (*Trichomonas vaginalis*) 20, 29–30, 153, 155
triploidy, fetal 132
trophoblast, extravillous 137–8
trophoblastic disease 128–35
  persistent 131–2
trophoblastic tumour, placental site 134–5
tuberculosis
  endometrial 53–5
  fallopian tube 81
tubo-ovarian abscess 79
twin pregnancy, placenta in 161–7
twin-to-twin transfusion syndrome 162

U
umbilical cord entanglement 162
urethral carcinoma 17
uterine sarcoma, undifferentiated 67
uteroplacental vessels, pathology of 137–8

V
vagina 19–24
  adenosis 20–2
  inflammation 19–20
  neoplasms 22–4
  vault/lateral wall smears 151, 167
vaginal intraepithelial neoplasia (VAIN) 21–2
vaginitis
  infective 19–20
  non-infective 19
  non-specific 19
verrucous carcinoma, vulva 16
villitis 139
VIN, *see* vulvar intraepithelial neoplasia
vulva 1–17
  benign tumours 11–12
  dermatological disorders 1–3
  dystrophies 1, 6
  inflammation 3–6
  malignant tumours 13–17
  non-invasive, intraepithelial neoplastic lesions 6–10
  non-neoplastic cysts 10–11
vulvar carcinoma
  invasive squamous cell 9, 13–15
    basaloid 14
    keratinising 13, 14
    warty (Bowenoid) 14
    verrucous 16
vulvar intraepithelial neoplasia (VIN) 6–9
  basaloid 7, 9
  Bowenoid 7, 8, 9, 14
  differentiated 8, 9
  undifferentiated 7–9
vulvitis
  infective 3–4
  non-infective 3

W
Walthard's rests 82
warts, *see* condylomata acuminata

Y
yolk sac tumours 115–16